KU-026-052

Department of Health
Welsh Office
Scottish Home and Health Department

IMMUNISATION
against
Infectious
Disease

1990

LONDON: HMSO

© *Crown copyright 1990*
First published 1990
ISBN 0 11 321251 8

Preface

The last edition of "Immunisation against Infectious Disease" represented a major revision of this Handbook. It was generally welcomed by those involved in immunisation practice and has helped to restore confidence in our national programme. Another important recent development was the appointment of Immunisation Co-ordinators in each Health District (with equivalent appointments in Northern Ireland, Scotland and Wales) which focused responsibility and accountability for immunisation at local level. The Joint Committee is grateful to the many individuals whose efforts are reflected in improved rates of immunisation and an encouraging fall in disease notifications, which in 1989 for measles were the lowest ever recorded. The continued cooperation of doctors in the prompt and accurate reporting of immunisation and notifiable infections is much appreciated.

This latest revision reflects the Joint Committee's wish to see the handbook updated regularly to keep pace with new developments. It contains several important changes, most notably the recommendation that infants are given earlier protection against whooping cough by accelerating the primary schedule. This change should also facilitate the more effective incorporation of immunisation into programmes of early child surveillance and improve the uptake in mobile families.

The BCG chapter describes the new packaging of the vaccine and more detailed guidance is given on the correct technique and site of vaccination. Careful tuberculin skin-testing is important, avoid the use of techniques or equipment that the Joint Committee does not recommend and pay scrupulous attention to the disinfection process (which is slightly modified in this issue).

Readers should also note that advice on immunoglobulins is now included in the relevant sections. Several parts have been re-written in continuing efforts to encourage positive attitudes towards achieving the maximum possible uptake of immunisation. Doctors are urged to follow these recommendations which are based on the current expert advice available to the Joint Committee, although in some circumstances they may differ from that contained in the vaccine manufacturers' data sheets.

Sections have been added on meningococcal infection and varicella zoster. It should be noted that the recently licensed meningococcal vaccine is now recommended, in addition to chemoprophylaxis, for close contacts of patients infected with groups A and C meningococci. There are appendices on Japanese B and Tick-borne encephalitis; and a rapid schedule of immunisation is provided for those travellers who have to go abroad at short notice.

In spite of the encouraging improvements of the last few years, a greater commitment to immunisation is still needed by all who work in the preventive services, if we are to reach our targets. A disturbing number of children are still being denied immunisation because of false contraindications. The exhortation included in Section 2.2 should be our watchword, "No child should be denied immunisation without serious thought to the consequences, both for the individual child and for the community".

I would like to record my gratitude and that of my colleagues on the Joint Committee to all who helped with the production of this handbook, but particularly to Dr David Salisbury and Dr Christine Miller as co-ordinators and editors, for the considerable time and effort put into this revision.

A G M Campbell MB, FRCP (Edin), DCH
Chairman Joint Committee on Vaccination and Immunisation
January 1990

The Joint Committee on Vaccination and Immunisation gratefully acknowledges the contributions to the Memorandum made by the BPA/JCVI Working Party, the Hepatitis Advisory Group, the BCG Subcommittee and the following individuals:-

Dr Joan Davies (Deputy Director, Public Health Laboratory Service)
Dr Sylvia Gardner (Virus Reference Laboratory, PHLS)
Dr Dennis Jones (Director, Manchester Public Health Laboratory)
Dr David Magrath (Head of Biologics, WHO, and formerly National Institute for Biological Standards and Control)
Dr Elizabeth Miller (Communicable Disease Surveillance Centre, PHLS)
Dr Nigel Peel (Director, Leeds PHL)
Dr Frank Sheffield (David Bruce Laboratory, and formerly NIBSC)
Dr J W G Smith (Director, PHLS)
Professor Richard Smithells (Emeritus Professor of Paediatrics and Child Health, University of Leeds)
Dr Bernard Rowe (Director, Division of Enteric Pathogens, PHLS)
Dr John Cradock-Watson (Public Health Laboratory)
Dr Susan Young (Deputy Director, CDSC)

Contents

Contents

* Routine programme
+ Adult/elective
# Travel

1   Introduction

1.1 Immunity can be induced, either actively or passively, against a variety of bacterial and viral agents.

1.2 **Active immunity** is induced by using inactivated or attenuated live organisms or their products. Live attenuated vaccines include those for poliomyelitis (OPV), measles and rubella, and BCG vaccine. Bacterial and viral vaccines such as whooping cough, typhoid and inactivated poliomyelitis (IPV) vaccines contain inactivated organisms.Others such as influenza and pneumococcal vaccine contain immunising components of the organisms; tetanus and diphtheria vaccines contain toxoid – that is, toxins inactivated by treatment with formaldehyde.

1.3 Most vaccines produce their protective effect by stimulating the production of antibodies which are detectable in the serum by laboratory tests. BCG vaccine promotes cell mediated immunity which is demonstrated by a positive tuberculin skin test.

1.4 A first injection of inactivated vaccine or toxoid in a subject without prior exposure to the antigen produces a slow antibody or antitoxin response of predominantly IgM antibody – the primary response. Two injections may be needed to produce such a response. Depending on the potency of the product and time interval, further injections will lead to an accelerated response in which the antibody or antitoxin titre (IgG) rises to a higher level – the secondary response. Following a full course, the antibody or antitoxin levels remain high for months or years, but even if the level of detectable antibody falls, the immune mechanism has been sensitised and a further dose of vaccine reinforces immunity.

1.5 Some inactivated vaccines contain adjuvants, substances which enhance the antibody response. Examples are aluminium phosphate and aluminium hydroxide which are contained in adsorbed diphtheria/tetanus/ pertussis vaccine, and adsorbed diphtheria/tetanus vaccine.

1.6 Live attenuated virus vaccines such as measles, rubella and mumps promote a full, long-lasting antibody response after one dose. Live poliomyelitis vaccine (OPV) requires three doses. An important additional

Immunisation against Infectious Disease   1

effect of poliomyelitis vaccine is the establishment of local immunity in the intestine.

1.7 **Passive immunity** results from the injection of human immunoglobulin (3.10); the protection afforded is immediate but lasts only for a few weeks. There are two types:

(i) Human normal immunoglobulin (HNIG) derived from the pooled plasma of donors and containing antibody to viruses which are currently prevalent in the general population. Examples of the use of HNIG are the protection of immunosuppressed children exposed to measles, and protection of individuals against hepatitis A.

(ii) Specific immunoglobulins for tetanus, hepatitis B, rabies and varicella/zoster. These are obtained from the pooled blood of convalescent patients, donors recently immunised with the relevant vaccine, or those who on screening are found to have sufficiently high antibody titres. Each specific immunoglobulin therefore contains antibody at a higher titre than that present in normal immunoglobulin.

1.8 Recommendations for the use of normal and specific immunoglobulins are given in the relevant sections.

2 General Topics

(i) Consent must be obtained (2.1), and suitability for immunisation established.

(ii) Doctors and nurses providing vaccination should have received training and be proficient in the appropriate techniques.

(iii) Preparations must be made for the management of anaphylaxis and other immediate reactions (see 3.8).

2.1 Consent

(i) Consent must always be obtained before immunisation.

(ii) Written consent provides a permanent record, but consent - either written or verbal - is required at the time of each immunisation after the child's fitness and suitability have been established (iv).

(iii) Consent obtained **before** the occasion upon which a child is brought for immunisation is only an agreement for the child to be included in the immunisation programme.

(iv) The bringing of a child for immunisation after an invitation to attend for this purpose may be viewed as acceptance that the child may be immunised. When a child is brought for this purpose and fitness and suitability have been established, consent to that immunisation may be implied in the absence of any expressed reservation to the immunisation proceeding at that stage. Similarly the attendance of a child at school on the day that the parent/guardian has been advised the child will be vaccinated may also be viewed as acceptance in the absence of any reservation expressed by the parent/guardian.

(v) If a child's fitness and suitability cannot be established, immunisation should be deferred.

2.2 Contraindications

Advice: No child should be denied immunisation without serious thought as to the consequences, both for the individual child and for the community. Where there is any doubt, advice should be sought from a Consultant Paediatrician, Specialist in Public Health

Immunisation against Infectious Disease

Medicine or District Immunisation Co-ordinator.

(i) Immunisation should be postponed if the subject is suffering from any acute illness. Minor infections in the absence of fever or systemic upset are not contraindications.

(ii) Although there is increasing evidence to suggest that rubella vaccine is not teratogenic (9.3.2), live vaccines should not be administered to pregnant women because of the theoretical possibility of harm to the fetus. Where there is a significant risk of exposure, for example to poliomyelitis or yellow fever, the need for vaccination outweighs any possible risk to the fetus.

(iii) Live vaccines should not be administered to the following; patients receiving high-dose corticosteroid (eg for children; prednisolone 2mg per kilogram per day for more than a week) or immunosuppressive treatment including general irradiation; those suffering from malignant conditions such as lymphoma, leukaemia, Hodgkin's disease or other tumours of the reticuloendothelial system; patients with impaired immunological mechanism as for example in hypogammaglobulinaemia. In adults, daily doses in excess of 60mg of prednisolone are associated with significant immunosuppression, although lower doses may be associated with some effect. Under such circumstances, live vaccines such as yellow fever vaccine or BCG should not be used; inactivated vaccines are not dangerous to the recipient but may be ineffective.

(iv) Individuals with immunosuppression from disease or chemotherapy (eg in remission from acute leukaemia), should not receive live virus vaccines until at least six months after chemotherapy has finished. Such patients and those in (iii) above), should be given in an injection of immunoglobulin as soon as possible after exposure to measles or chickenpox (see Sections 8 and 21).

(v) For individuals treated with systemic corticosteroids at high dose (for children; prednisolone 2mg/kg/day for more than a week; for adults as in (iii) above), live vaccines should be postponed until at least three months after treatment has stopped. Children on lower daily doses of systemic corticosteroids for less than two weeks, and those on lower doses on alternate day regimens for longer periods, may be given live virus vaccines.

(vi) Live virus vaccines, with the exception of yellow fever vaccine, should not be given during the three months following injection of immunoglobulin because the immune response may be inhibited. Normal human immunoglobulin obtained from UK residents is unlikely

Immunisation against Infectious Disease

to contain antibody to yellow fever virus which would inactivate the vaccine.

(vii) For HIV-positive individuals, see 2.4.

Specific contraindications to individual vaccines are given in the relevant sections and must be observed.

2.2.1 The following conditions are NOT contraindications to vaccination:-

a. Asthma, eczema, hay fever or 'snuffles'.
b. Treatment with antibiotics or locally-acting (eg topical or inhaled) steroids.
c. Mother pregnant.
d. Child being breast fed.
e. History of jaundice after birth.
f. Under a certain weight.
g. Over the age given in immunisation schedule.
h. Previous history of pertussis, measles, rubella or mumps infection.
i. Prematurity: immunisation should not be postponed.
j. Stable neurological conditions such as cerebral palsy and Down's syndrome.
k. Contact with an infectious disease.
l. Homœopathy: the Council of the Faculty of Homœopathy strongly supports the vaccination programme and has stated that vaccination should be carried out in the normal way using the conventional tested and approved vaccines, in the absence of medical contraindications.

2.2.2 A history of allergy is NOT a contraindication. Hypersensitivity to egg contraindicates influenza vaccine; previous **anaphylactic** reaction to egg contraindicates measles, mumps, rubella, influenza and yellow fever vaccines.

2.2.3 Siblings and close contacts of immunosuppressed children **should** be immunised against measles, mumps and rubella. There is no risk of transmission of virus following vaccination.

2.2.4 Oral poliomyelitis vaccine (OPV) should **not** be given to immunosuppressed children, their siblings or other household contacts. Inactivated poliomyelitis vaccine should be given instead; this should also be given to immunosuppressed adults and their contacts (see 7.3.9).

Immunisation against Infectious Disease   5

2.3 Special risk groups

2.3.1 Some conditions increase the risk from infectious diseases and children with such conditions should be vaccinated as a matter of priority. These conditions include the following:- asthma, chronic lung and congenital heart diseases, Down's syndrome, antibody-positive to the Human Immunodeficiency Virus (HIV, 2.4), small for dates and born prematurely. This last group should be immunised according to the recommended schedule from two months after birth, irrespective of the extent of prematurity.

2.3.2 If it is necessary to administer more than one live virus vaccine at the same time, they should either be given simultaneously in different sites (unless a combined preparation is used) or be separated by a period of at least three weeks. It is also recommended that a three week interval should be allowed between the administration of live virus vaccines and BCG vaccine.

2.4 Immunisation of individuals with antibody to the Human Immunodeficiency Virus (HIV positive)

2.4.1 HIV positive individuals, **WITH OR WITHOUT SYMPTOMS SHOULD**, receive the following as appropriate;

Live vaccines: **measles: mumps: rubella: polio:**

Inactivated vaccines: **whooping cough: diphtheria: tetanus: polio: typhoid: cholera: hepatitis B.**

2.4.2 For HIV-positive symptomatic individuals, inactivated polio vaccine (IPV) may be used instead of OPV, at the discretion of the clinician.

2.4.3 HIV-positive individuals should NOT receive **BCG** vaccine; there have been reports of dissemination of BCG in HIV positive individuals.

2.4.4 Yellow fever vaccine should not be given to either symptomatic or asymptomatic HIV-positive individuals since there is as yet insufficient evidence as to the safety of its use. Travellers should be told of this uncertainty and advised not to be vaccinated unless there are compelling reasons.

2.4.5 No harmful effects have been reported following live attenuated vaccines for **measles, mumps, rubella and polio** in HIV positive individuals who are at increased risk from these diseases. It should be noted that in HIV positive individuals, polio virus may be excreted for longer periods than in normal persons. Contacts of a recently vaccinated HIV positive individual should be warned of this, and of the need for washing their hands after changing a vaccinated infant's nappies. For HIV positive contacts of a vaccinated individual (whether that individual is HIV positive or not) the potential risk of infection is greater than that in normal individuals.

2.4.6 Vaccine efficacy may be reduced in HIV positive individuals. Consideration should be given to the use of normal immunoglobulin for HIV positive individuals after exposure to measles (8.7).

2.4.7 For HIV positive individuals exposed to **chickenpox or zoster,** see 21.5.

NB. SOME OF THE ABOVE ADVICE DIFFERS FROM THAT FOR OTHER IMMUNOCOMPROMISED PATIENTS (2.2).

2.5 Surveillance and reporting of suspected adverse reactions

2.5.1 All vaccines are extensively tested for safety and efficacy before licensing, but careful surveillance must be maintained. This depends on early, complete and accurate reporting of suspected adverse reactions to the Committee on Safety of Medicines, using the yellow card system. **Serious** suspected reactions, including those which are fatal, life-threatening, disabling, incapacitating or which result in hospitalisation **must** be reported; this applies to all serious reactions whether or not such reactions have been previously recognised.

2.5.2 Yellow cards are supplied to general practitioners and pharmacists, and are available from the Committee on Safety of Medicines, 1 Nine Elms Lane, London SW8 5NQ. They are also available as pages of the British National Formulary number 13 (1987) onwards.

3 Immunisation Procedures

3.1 Preliminary points

3.1.1 Before administering any immunological product, attention should be paid to the following points:

a. The leaflets supplied with the product and prepared by the manufacturer in consultation with the Licensing Authority should be read (but see Preface).

b. The identity of the vaccine must be checked to ensure the right product is used in the appropriate way on every occasion.

c. The expiry date must be noted.

d. The date of vaccination, title of vaccine and batch number must be recorded on the recipient's record. When two vaccines are given simultaneously, the relevant sites should be recorded to allow any reactions to be related to the causative vaccine.

e. The recommended storage conditions must have been observed (see 3.9).

3.2 Reconstitution of vaccines

3.2.1 Freeze dried vaccines must be reconstituted with the diluent supplied and used within the recommended period after reconstitution (see 3.8.2).

3.2.2 Before injection, the colour of the product must be checked with that stated by the manufacturer in the package insert. The diluent should be added slowly to avoid frothing. A sterile 1ml syringe with a 21G needle should be used for reconstituting the vaccine, and a small gauge needle for injection (see 3.5).

3.3 Cleaning of skin

3.3.1 The skin should be cleaned with a suitable preparation (eg mediswabs containing alcohol only). Alcohol and other disinfecting agents must be allowed to evaporate before injection of vaccine since they can inactivate live vaccine preparations.

3.4 Route of administration

(i) By mouth

Oral polio vaccine must NEVER be injected. Sugar lumps, if used, should be prepared with OPV immediately before administration; allowing them to stand at room temperature for any length of time may decrease the potency of the vaccine.

(ii) Subcutaneous and intramuscular injection

With the exception of BCG and OPV, all vaccines should be given by intramuscular or deep subcutaneous injection. In infants, the antero-lateral aspect of the thigh or upper arm are recommended. If the buttock is used, injection into the upper outer quadrant avoids the risk of sciatic nerve damage. Injection into fatty tissue of the buttock has been shown to reduce the efficacy of hepatitis B vaccine.

(iii) Intradermal injections

BCG vaccine is ALWAYS given intradermally; rabies vaccine may also be given this way. When giving an intradermal injection, the operator should stretch the skin between the thumb and forefinger of one hand, and with the other slowly insert the needle (size 25G), bevel upwards, for about 2mm into the superficial layers of the dermis, almost parallel with the surface. A raised, blanched bleb showing the tips of the hair follicles is a sign that the injection has been made correctly and its diameter gives a useful indication of the amount that has been injected. Considerable resistance is felt from a correctly given intradermal injection. If this is not felt, and it is suspected that the needle is too deep, it should be removed and reinserted before more vaccine is given. A bleb of 7mm diameter is approximately equivalent to 0.1ml.

(iv) Suitable sites for intradermal injections

  a. For BCG the site of injection is over the insertion of the left deltoid muscle; the tip of the shoulder must be avoided because of the increased risk of keloid formation at this site (see 10.3).

   b. For tuberculin sensitivity tests (Mantoux or Heaf), intradermal injections are given in the middle of the flexor surface of the forearm. This site should not be used for injecting vaccines.

   c. The use of jet injectors is NOT recommended.

   d. For intradermal rabies vaccine, the site of injection is behind the posterior border of the distal portion of the deltoid muscle.

3.5 Administration

Vaccine	Route of administration	Dose	Needle size
OPV	Oral	3 drops	Nil
IPV	Deep subcutaneous or intramuscular	0.5ml	23G
DPT) DT)	Deep subcutaneous or intramuscular	0.5ml	23G
Measles) Mumps) Rubella)	Deep subcutaneous or intramuscular	0.5ml	23G
Typhoid	Deep subcutaneous or intramuscular	0.5ml	23G
BCG	Intradermal Infants	0.1ml 0.05ml	25G
Rabies	Deep subcutaneous or intramuscular	1.0ml	23G
	Intradermal	0.1ml	25G
Anthrax	Deep subcutaneous or intramuscular	0.5ml	23G
Hepatitis B	Deep subcutaneous or intramuscular	1.0ml	23G

3.6 Schedule

3.6.1 **The schedule for primary immunisation with DPT and polio has been changed to start at two months, with an interval of one month between each dose. In Scotland, the schedule for primary immunisation starts at 2 months and must be completed by six months with intervals between injections of not less than one month. This will allow for the completion of the primary course at an earlier age, to provide protection against whooping cough for the youngest children for whom it is most dangerous. No booster dose of pertussis vaccine will be required; the fourth D/T polio booster will continue to be given before school entry.**

3.6.2 The change has been made following recognition that one of the most frequent reasons for low vaccine uptake is the mobility of young families who move out of districts before their children have completed primary courses. This problem is compounded by the variation in schedules between Health Authorities. The new schedule at two, three and four months will remove this problem by providing uniformity; starting the programme earlier and shortening the intervals will reduce the opportunities for failing to complete a course.

3.6.3 Children who commence the accelerated immunisation schedule should receive their primary immunisations at one month intervals. Children who have already started the primary course should receive the remaining doses at one month intervals.

3.6.4 The rationale for the previous extended intervals between doses was a possibly improved immunogenic response; this was at a time (1968) when the potency of pertussis vaccine was in question. However, recent studies comparing the antibody levels of diphtheria, pertussis, tetanus and poliomyelitis one year after the third dose showed them to be similar for both accelerated and extended schedules.

3.6.5 Studies are being undertaken to monitor levels of immunity and adverse events associated with the new schedule.

3.6.6 Every effort should be made to ensure that **all children are vaccinated even if they are younger or older than the recommended age-range; no opportunity to immunise should be missed.**

3.6.7 When such opportunistic immunisation has been carried out, it must be reported to the Health Authority (HA) or Family Practitioner Committee (FPC) as an unscheduled immunisation.

3.6.8 If any course of immunisation is interrupted it should be resumed and completed as soon as possible, but not repeated.

3.6.9 The schedule for routine immunisation is given below. Details of procedure for each vaccine are given in the relevant sections and should be consulted.

Vaccine		Age	Notes
D/T/P and polio	1st dose	2 months	)
	2nd dose	3 months	) Primary Course*
	3rd dose	4 months	)
Measles/mumps/ rubella (MMR)		12-18 months	Can be given at any age over 12 months
Booster D/T and polio		4-5 years	
Rubella		10-14 years	GIRLS ONLY
BCG		10-14 years or infancy	Interval of 3 weeks between BCG and rubella
Booster tetanus and polio		15-18 years	

*For Scotland, see para. 3.6.1.

CHILDREN should therefore have received the following vaccines:

By 6 months: 3 doses of DTP and polio, or DT and polio.
By 18 months: measles/mumps/rubella.
By school entry: 4th DT and polio; measles/mumps/rubella if missed earlier.

Between 10 and 14 years: BCG; rubella for girls.
Before leaving school: 5th polio and tetanus.

ADULTS should receive the following vaccines:

Women sero-negative for rubella: rubella.
Previously unimmunised individuals: polio, tetanus.
Individuals in high risk groups: hepatitis B, influenza.

3.7 Immunisation by nurses

A doctor may delegate responsibility for immunisation to a nurse provided the following conditions are fulfilled:

(i) The nurse is willing to be professionally accountable for this work.
(ii) The nurse has received training and is competent in all aspects of immunisation, including the contraindications to specific vaccines.
(iii) Adequate training has been given in the recognition and treatment of anaphylaxis.

If these conditions are fulfilled and nurses carry out the immunisation in accordance with accepted District Health Authority policy, the Authority will accept responsibility for immunisation by nurses.

3.8 Anaphylaxis

3.8.1 Recipients of vaccine should remain under observation until they have been seen to recover from the procedure. It is not possible to specify an exact length of time.

3.8.2 **In the period 1978-89, 118 anaphylactic and anaphylactoid reactions following vaccinations were reported to the Committee on Safety of Medicines; no deaths were reported. Furthermore, during this time no deaths from this cause were notified to the Office of Population, Censuses and Surveys (OPCS). During the period, approximately 25 million childhood vaccinations were given.** Anaphylactic reactions are thus very rare, but they are also unexpected and can be fatal. Any individual carrying out immunisation procedures must therefore be able to distinguish between anaphylaxis, convulsions, and fainting. The last is relatively common after immunisation of adults and adolescents; very young children rarely faint and sudden loss of consciousness at this age should be presumed to be an anaphylactic reaction **in the absence of a strong central pulse (ie carotid), which**

Immunisation against Infectious Disease   13

persists during a faint or convulsion.

3.8.3 The following symptoms may develop:

a. Pallor, limpness and apnoea are the commonest signs in children.

b. Upper airway obstruction; hoarseness and stridor as a result of angio-oedema involving hypopharynx, epiglottis and larynx.

c. Lower airway obstruction; subjective feelings of retrosternal tightness and dyspnoea with audible expiratory wheeze from bronchospasm.

d. Cardiovascular; sinus tachycardia, profound hypotension in association with tachycardia; severe bradycardia.

e. Skin; characteristic rapid development of urticarial lesions–circumscribed, intensely itchy weals with erythematous raised edges and pale blanched centres.

3.8.4 Management

Such events happen without warning. Adrenaline and appropriate sized oral airways must therefore always be immediately at hand whenever immunisation is given. **All doctors and nurses responsible for immunisation must be familiar with the practical steps necessary to save life following an anaphylactic reaction.**

a. Lie patient in left lateral position. If unconscious, insert airway.

b. Give 1/1000 adrenaline by deep intramuscular injection **unless there is a strong central pulse and the patient's condition is good.** See Table below for dosage.

c. If oxygen is available, give it by face mask.

d. Send for professional assistance. NEVER LEAVE PATIENT ALONE.

e. If appropriate, begin cardio-pulmonary resuscitation.

f. Chlorpheniramine maleate (piriton) 2.5-5mg may be given **intravenously,** by appropriately trained individuals. Hydrocortisone (100mg intravenously) may also be given to prevent further deterioration in severely affected cases.

g. If there is no improvement in the patient's condition in ten minutes, repeat the dose of adrenaline up to a maximum of three doses.

h. All cases should be admitted to hospital for observation.

i. The reaction should be reported to the Committee on Safety of Medicines using the yellow card system.

Immunisation against Infectious Disease

3.8.5 **Adrenaline dosage**   Adrenaline 1/1000 (1mg/ml)

Adults: 0.5 to 1.0ml repeated as necessary up to a maximum of three doses.
The lower dose should be used for the elderly or those of slight build.

Infants and children:

Age	Dose of adrenaline
Less than 1 year	0.05ml
1 year	0.1ml
2 years	0.2ml
3-4 years	0.3ml
5 years	0.4ml
6-10 years	0.5ml

3.9 Storage and disposal of vaccines

3.9.1 Manufacturers' recommendations on storage must be observed and
care should be taken to ensure that, on receipt, vaccines are immediately
placed under the required storage conditions. Vaccines must not be kept at
temperatures below 0°C as freezing can cause the deterioration of the
vaccine and breakage of the container.

3.9.2 A pharmacist or other suitably trained person should be nominated
for each clinic as being responsible for the safe storage of vaccines, and
should work to a written procedure developed to meet local needs. This
person should have a designated deputy to cover in times of absence.

3.9.3 A maximum/minimum thermometer should be used in refrigerators
where vaccines are stored, irrespective of whether the refrigerator
incorporates a temperature indicator dial. Such thermometers may be
purchased from reputable laboratory suppliers, some of whom are able to
provide a certificate of conformance/calibration.

3.9.4 The maximum and minimum temperatures reached should be
monitored and recorded regularly and at least at the beginning of each
vaccination session. The written procedure referred to in 3.9.2 should
indicate the action to be taken in the event of the temperature going
outwith the specified range.

Immunisation against Infectious Disease   15

3.9.5 Special care should be taken during defrosting to ensure that the temperature of the vaccine does not exceed the specified range for significant periods of time. An alternative refrigerator or insulated containers should be used for vaccine.

3.9.6 Reconstituted vaccine must be used within the recommended period, varying from one to four hours, according to the manufacturer's instructions. Single dose containers are preferable; once opened, multi-dose vials must not be kept after the end of the session and any vaccine left unused must be discarded.

3.9.7 Further information and a fact sheet on refrigeration equipment and accessories are available from: Supplies Technology Division, Product Group 1B, 14 Russell Square, London WC1B 5EP. Tel. No. 071-636 6811 Ext. 3059 or 3048.

3.9.8 Unused vaccine, spent or partly spent vials, should be disposed of safely, preferably by heat inactivation or incineration. Contaminated waste and spillage should be dealt with by heat sterilisation, incineration or chemical disinfection as appropriate. Those providing live vaccines should consult their local Control of Infection Committee about suitable procedures.

3.10 **Immunoglobulin** (and see under relevant Sections)

3.10.1 All immunoglobulins are prepared from the blood of donors who are negative to hepatitis B (HBsAg) and human immunodeficiency virus (HIV).

3.10.2 *Human Normal Immunoglobulin (HNIG)*

This is prepared from the pooled plasma of blood donors and contains antibody to measles, varicella, hepatitis A and other viruses which are currently prevalent in the population. Immunoglobulin prepared by Blood Products Laboratory and supplied through PHLS is available in 1.7ml ampoules containing 250mg, and 5ml ampoules containing 750mg. It is given by intramuscular injection. It must be stored at 0-4°C and the expiry date on the packet must be observed. It has a shelf life of three years when correctly stored. Unused portions of an ampoule must be discarded. Commercial products are also available.

Immunisation against Infectious Disease

3.10.3 Recommendations for the use of HNIG for prophylaxis of measles and hepatitis A are given in 8.7.1 and 12.3 respectively. It is not recommended for prevention of mumps (8.7.2) or rubella (8.7.3).

3.10.4 HNIG may interfere with the immune response to live virus vaccines which should therefore be given at least three weeks before or three months after an injection of HNIG. This does not apply to yellow fever vaccine since HNIG obtained from donors in the UK is unlikely to contain antibody to this virus. For travellers abroad this interval may not be possible, but in the case of live polio vaccine, this is likely to be a booster dose for which the possible inhibiting effect of HNIG is less important.

3.10.5 *Supplies*

Central Public Health Laboratory Tel. 081 200 6868
Public Health Laboratories, England and Wales
Blood Transfusion Service, Scotland
Blood Products Laboratory Tel. 081 953 6191
The Laboratories, Belfast City Hospital. Tel. 0232 329341

Immuno. Tel. 0732 458101 (Gammabulin)
Kabivitrum. Tel. 0895 51144 (Kabiglobulin)

3.10.6 *Specific Immunoglobulins*

These are available for tetanus, hepatitis B, rabies and varicella/zoster. They are prepared from the pooled plasma of blood donors who have a recent history of infection or vaccination, or who on screening are found to have suitably high titres of antibody. Recommendations for their use are given in the relevant Sections: tetanus (6.3.4); hepatitis B (13.8); rabies (14.7); varicella/zoster (21.3 - 21.11).

Anti-tetanus immunoglobulin
  Regional Blood Transfusion Centres
  Wellcome. Tel. 0270 583151 (Humotet)
  Scotland; Blood Transfusion Service

Anti-hepatitis B immunoglobulin
  Communicable Disease Surveillance Centre Tel. 081 200 6868
  Public Health Laboratories, England and Wales
  Scotland; Blood Transfusion Service (13.8)
  Regional Virus Laboratory, Royal Victoria Hospital, Belfast Tel. 0232
  240503
  Biotest (UK) Ltd. Tel. 021 733 3393

Anti-rabies immunoglobulin
  Central Public Health Laboratory (Virus Reference Laboratory)
  Tel. 081 200 6868
  The Laboratories, Belfast City Hospital, Tel. 0232 329241
  Scotland; Blood Transfusion Service

Anti-Varicella/zoster immunoglobulin
  Communicable Disease Surveillance Centre. Tel. 081 200 6868
  Public Health Laboratories, England and Wales
  Blood Products Laboratory Tel. 081 953 6191
  The Laboratories, Belfast City Hospital Tel. 0232 329241
  Scotland; Blood Transfusion Service
  Biotest (UK) Ltd. Tel. 021 733 3393

3.11 BIBLIOGRAPHY

Immunisation for the immunosuppressed child.
Campbell A G M.
Arch. Dis. Childhood 1988: 63(2); 113-4.

Human Immunodeficiency Virus infection and routine childhood
immunisation.
von Reyn C F, Clements C J, Mann J M.
The Lancet 1987: ii: 669.

Global Programme on AIDS and Expanded Programme on Immunisation. Joint WHO/UNICEF statement on early immunisation for HIV-infected children.
Weekly Epidem. Rec. 1989 No 7. (Feb. 17); 48-49.

Immunization of Children infected with Human Immunodeficiency Virus: supplementary ACIP statement.
MMWR 1988; 37 (12); 181-5.

The efficacy of DPT and oral poliomyelitis immunisation schedules initiated from birth to 12 weeks of age.
Halsey N, Galazka A.
Bulletin of World Health Organisation 1985: 63 (6); 1151-69.

Durability of immunity to diphtheria, tetanus and poliomyelitis after a three dose immunisation schedule completed in the first eight months of life.
Jones A E, Johns A, Magrath D I, Melville-Smith M, Sheffield F.
Vaccine 1989: 7; 300-302.

The safe disposal of clinical waste.
Health and Safety Commission: Health Services Advisory Committee, 1982.
HMSO ISBN 0 11 883641 2.

4   Whooping Cough (Pertussis)

4.1 Introduction

4.1.1 Whooping cough is a highly infectious bacterial disease caused by *Bordetella pertussis* and spread by droplet infection; the incubation period is seven to ten days. A case is infectious from seven days after exposure to three weeks after the onset of typical paroxysms. The initial catarrhal stage has an insidious onset and is the most infectious period. An irritating cough gradually becomes paroxysmal, usually within one to two weeks, and often lasts for two to three months. In young infants, the typical "whoop" may never develop and coughing spasms may be followed by periods of apnoea. Whooping cough may be complicated by bronchopneumonia, repeated post-tussive vomiting leading to weight loss, and by cerebral hypoxia with a resulting risk of brain damage. Severe complications and deaths occur most commonly in infants under six months of age.

4.1.2 Before the large scale introduction of pertussis vaccination in the 1950's, the average annual number of notifications in England and Wales (E and W) exceeded 100,000. By 1973, when vaccine acceptance was over 80%, annual notifications of whooping cough had fallen to around 2,400.

4.1.3 Because of public anxiety about the safety and efficacy of the vaccine, acceptance rates fell to about 30% in 1975 and major epidemics with over 100,000 notified cases followed (in E and W) in 1977/79 and 1981/83. However increased vaccine uptake resulting from the return of public confidence cut short the next epidemic which died away in 1986, well below the levels of the previous two. In 1988 uptake of vaccine reached 73% and only 5027 cases were notified, the lowest number since the early 1970's.

4.1.4 Until the mid 1970's, mortality from whooping cough was about one per 1000 notified cases with a higher rate for infants under one year. In 1978 however when there were over 65,000 notifications (in E and W), only 12 deaths were notified. The actual number of deaths due to whooping cough is undoubtedly higher since not all cases in infants are recognised.

Graph 1

Whooping Cough Notifications (E&W)
Source: OPCS

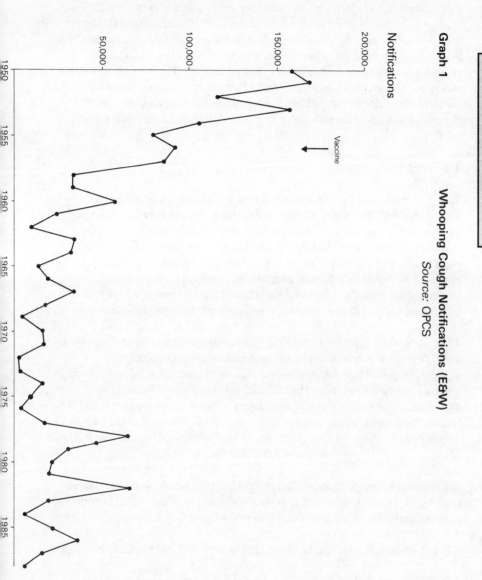

4.1.5 Since the anxieties concerning pertussis vaccine in the mid 1970s, studies have confirmed that a full course of vaccine confers protection in over 80% of recipients; in those not fully protected the disease is usually less severe. The two large epidemics which followed the reduction in vaccine acceptance are additional evidence of the effectiveness of pertussis vaccine in the prevention of disease. In Regions with particularly low vaccine acceptance rates, whooping cough notifications in 1986 were significantly higher than those in Regions with high acceptance rates.

4.2 Vaccine

4.2.1 Pertussis vaccine is a suspension of killed *Bordetella pertussis* organisms with an estimated potency of not less than four International Units in each 0.5ml of vaccine. The vaccine is usually given as a triple vaccine combined with diphtheria and tetanus vaccines, with an adjuvant such as aluminium hydroxide (DTPer/Vac/Ads, Trivax Ads). It is also available without the adjuvant as plain DTPer/Vac, and as a monovalent pertussis vaccine. The adsorbed vaccine should be used as it is more immunogenic and causes fewer systemic reactions, especially fever.

4.2.2 Adsorbed diphtheria/tetanus/pertussis vaccine (DTPer/Vac/Ads): one 0.5ml dose consists of a mixture in isotonic buffer solution of diphtheria toxoid and tetanus toxoid adsorbed on to aluminium hydroxide gel, together with not more than 20,000 million *Bordetella pertussis* organisms. The potency of the diphtheria component is not less than 30 Iu; that of the tetanus component not less than 60 Iu and that of the pertussis component not less than an estimated 4 Iu. Thiomersal is added as a preservative to a final concentration of 0.01%.

4.2.3 Monovalent pertussis vaccine: one 0.5ml dose contains not more than 20,000 million *Bordetella pertussis* organisms. Thiomersal is added as a preservative to a final concentration of 0.01%.

4.2.4 The vaccines should be stored betweed 2-8°C, but not frozen.

4.2.5 The dose is 0.5ml given by deep subcutaneous or intramuscular injection.

4.3 Recommendations

4.3.1 Adsorbed pertussis vaccine as a component of the primary course of immunisation against diphtheria, tetanus and pertussis (DTPer/Vac/Ads) is recommended for all infants from two months of age, unless there is a genuine contraindication (see 4.5).

4.3.2 The primary course consists of **three doses with an interval of one month between each dose** (see 3.6). If the primary course is interrupted it should be resumed but not repeated, allowing appropriate intervals between the remaining doses.

4.3.3 Monovalent pertussis vaccine can be given when the pertussis component has been omitted from earlier vaccinations. Children who have received a full course of vaccination against diphtheria and tetanus should be given three doses of monovalent pertussis vaccine at monthly intervals.

4.3.4 Where the primary course of diphtheria/tetanus immunisation has been started and the parent wishes pertussis vaccine to be added, DTP vaccine may be used for the subsequent doses, followed by monovalent pertussis vaccine at monthly intervals to complete the three doses. Similarly, children presenting for their pre-school diphtheria/tetanus booster who have not previously been immunised against pertussis should be given triple vaccine as the first dose, with two subsequent doses of monovalent pertussis vaccine at monthly intervals.

4.3.5 The low uptake of pertussis vaccine from 1975-1985 left a considerable number of unimmunised older children who received DT vaccine only. Such children should be immunised with single antigen pertussis vaccine, both for their own protection and for that of young siblings under the age of vaccination; **there is no upper age limit.**

4.3.6 No reinforcing dose of pertussis vaccine is necessary after a course of three injections.

4.3.7 If pertussis vaccine is contraindicated or refused by parents, then DT/Vac/Ads should be offered.

4.3.8 HIV-positive individuals may receive pertussis vaccine in the absence of contraindications given in 4.5.

Immunisation against Infectious Disease 23

Whooping Cough

4.4 Adverse reactions

4.4.1 a. Swelling and redness at the injection site are common (see 4.5.1b). A small painless nodule may form at the injection site which usually disappears and is of no consequence.

b. Crying, screaming and fever may occur after pertussis vaccine in triple vaccine; they may also occur after vaccine which does not contain the pertussis component. Attacks of high pitched screaming, episodes of pallor, cyanosis, limpness, convulsions, as well as local reactions have been reported after both adsorbed DTP and DT vaccines. Both local and systemic reactions are more common after the plain preparations which do not contain adjuvant.

c. More severe neurological conditions, including encephalopathy and prolonged convulsions, resulting in permanent brain damage and death, have been reported after pertussis vaccine. But such illnesses can develop from a variety of causes in the first year of life in both vaccinated and unvaccinated children and there is no specific test which can identify cases which may be caused by pertussis vaccine. Therefore, no wholly reliable estimate of the risk of such complications due to the vaccine can be made.

d. For these reasons, considerable public and professional anxiety persists on the safety of pertussis vaccine. In Great Britain, between 1976 and 1979, a total of 1182 children with serious acute neurological illnesses were reported to the National Childhood Encephalopathy Study (NCES). Only 39 of these children had recently had pertussis vaccine and in many of these, the association of the neurological illnesses with vaccination could have occurred by chance. Analysis of the results showed that, after taking this into account, the vaccine may very rarely be associated with the development of severe acute neurological illness in children who were previously apparently normal; most of these children suffered no apparent harm. **The number of cases in the NCES, even after three years of intensive case finding, was too small to show conclusively whether or not the vaccine can cause permanent brain damage if such damage occurs at all.**

e. In the USA a group of children who had had convulsions or hypotonic-hyporesponsive episodes within 48 hours of DTP were reviewed six to seven years later; there was no evidence of serious neurological damage or intellectual impairment as a result of these episodes. In another American study, while an association was demonstrated between the first febrile convulsion and the scheduled age of pertussis immunisation, no

Immunisation against Infectious Disease

relationship was demonstrated between immunisation and the age of onset of epilepsy.

f. Neurological complications after whooping cough disease are considerably more common than after vaccine

g. Cot deaths (sudden infant death syndrome) occur most commonly during the first year of life and may therefore coincide with the giving of DTP vaccine. However studies have established that this association is temporal rather than causal.

4.4.2 If a febrile convulsion occurs after a dose of triple vaccine, specialist advice should be sought before continuing with any immunisation.

4.4.3 When pertussis vaccine is genuinely contraindicated, immunisation against diphtheria and tetanus should still be considered.

4.4.4 Severe reactions to whooping cough vaccine must be reported to the Committee on Safety of Medicines using the yellow card system.

4.5 Contraindications to pertussis immunisation

4.5.1 a. If the child is suffering from any acute illness, immunisation should be postponed until it has fully recovered. Minor infections without fever or systemic upset are not reasons to postpone immunisation.

b. Immunisation should not be carried out in children who have a history of severe local or general reaction to a preceding dose. The following reactions should be regarded as severe:-

Local: an extensive area of redness and swelling which becomes indurated and involves most of the antero-lateral surface of the thigh or a major part of the circumference of the upper arm. This reaction may increase in severity with each subsequent injection.

General: fever equal to or more than 39.5 °C within 48 hours of vaccine; anaphylaxis; bronchospasm; laryngeal oedema; generalised collapse; prolonged unresponsiveness; prolonged inconsolable screaming; convulsions occurring within 72 hours.

4.5.2 A personal or family history of allergy is NOT a contraindication to immunisation against whooping cough, nor are stable neurological

Immunisation against Infectious Disease   25

conditions such as cerebral palsy or spina bifida. Children with evolving neurological conditions may be immunised later when the condition has become stable. For other false "contraindications" see 2.2.1.

4.6 Children with problem histories

There are certain groups of children in whom the advisability of whooping cough immunisation requires special consideration because of their own or their family histories. For these children, the likelihood of febrile convulsions following vaccine may be higher, but the effects of whooping cough disease could be more severe. The balance of risk and benefit should be assessed in each case. **Where there is doubt, appropriate advice should be sought from a consultant paediatrician, District Immunisation Co-ordinator or Specialist in Public Health Medicine rather than withholding vaccine, as many children in the following groups can be given pertussis vaccine. When pertussis vaccine is given to such children, parents should be given advice on the management of pyrexia and the prevention of febrile convulsions.**

These groups are:

(i) Children with a documented history of cerebral damage in the neonatal period; discharge summaries from neonatal units should identify such children and state whether or not pertussis vaccine should be given.
(ii) Children with a personal history of convulsions.
(iii) Children whose parents or siblings have a history of idiopathic epilepsy. In such children there may be a risk of developing a similar condition irrespective of vaccine.

4.7 Management of outbreaks

Since a course of three injections is required to protect against whooping cough, vaccine cannot be used to control an outbreak.

4.8 Supplies

All pertussis vaccines are manufactured and supplied by the Wellcome Foundation Ltd. Tel. Crewe (0270) 583151.

Immunisation against Infectious Disease

4.9 Bibliography

Infants and children with convulsions and hypotonic/hyporesponsive episodes following DTP immunisation; follow-up evaluation.
Barraff L J, Shields W D et al.
Pediatrics 1988; 81; 789-794.

Relationship of pertussis immunisation to the onset of neurological disorders: a retrospective epidemiological study.
Shields W D, Nielson C et al.
J. Pediatrics 1988: 81; 801-805.

Vaccination and cot deaths in perspective.
Roberts S C .
Arch. Dis. Child. 1987: 12; 754-9.

DHSS Whooping Cough: Reports from the Committee on Safety of Medicines and the Joint Committee on Vaccination and Immunisation.
HMSO 1981.

Severity of notified whooping cough.
Miller C L and Fletcher W B.
BMJ 1976, (1), 117-119.

Pertussis immunisation and serious acute neurological illness in children.
Miller D L, Ross E M, Alderslade R, Bellman M H, Rawson NSB.
BMJ 1981: 282; 1595-1599.

Symptoms after primary immunisation with DTP and with DT vaccine.
Pollock T M, Miller E, Mortimer J Y, Smith G.
Lancet 1984: ii; 146-149.

Efficacy of pertussis vaccination in England.
PHLS Epidemiological Research Laboratory and 21 Area Health Authorities.
BMJ 1982: 285; 357-359.

Communicable Disease Report Oct-Dec 1986.
Community Medicine 1987: 9; 176-181.

5 Diphtheria

5.1 Introduction

5.1.1 Diphtheria is an acute infectious disease affecting the upper respiratory tract and occasionally the skin. It is characterised by an inflammatory exudate which forms a greyish membrane in the respiratory tract which may cause obstruction. The incubation period is from two to five days. The disease is communicable for up to four weeks, but carriers may shed organisms for longer. A toxin is produced by diphtheria bacilli which affects particularly myocardium and nervous and adrenal tissues. Spread is by droplet infection and through contact with articles soiled by infected persons (fomites).

5.1.2 Effective protection against the disease is provided by active immunisation. The introduction of immunisation against diphtheria on a national scale in 1940 resulted in a dramatic fall in the number of notified cases and deaths from the disease. In 1940, 46,281 cases with 2,480 deaths were notified, compared with 37 cases and six deaths in 1957. From 1979 to 1988, 31 cases were notified with only one death.

See Graph ii Page 29

5.1.3 The disease and the organism have been virtually eliminated from the United Kingdom; the few cases which have occurred in recent years have nearly all been imported. There is thus no possibility now of acquiring natural immunisation from subclinical infection. A high vaccine acceptance rate must therefore be maintained in order to protect the population against the possibility of a resurgence of the disease which could follow the introduction of cases from overseas.

5.2 Diphtheria vaccine

5.2.1 Diphtheria immunisation protects by stimulating the production of antitoxin which provides immunity to the effects of the toxin. The immunogen is prepared by treating a cell-free purified preparation of toxin with formaldehyde, thereby converting it into the innocuous diphtheria

Graph 2

Diphtheria Notifications (E&W)
Source: OPCS

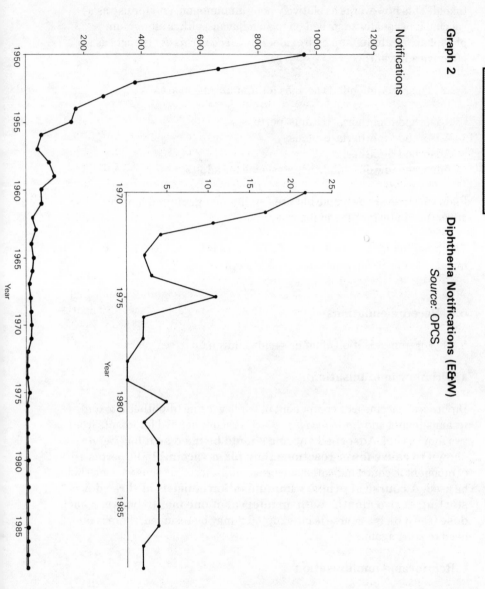

toxoid. This however is a relatively poor immunogen, and for use as a vaccine it is usually adsorbed on to an adjuvant, either aluminium phosphate or aluminium hydroxide. *Bordetella pertussis* also acts as an effective adjuvant.

5.2.2 The recommended vaccines for immunisation are:-

Adsorbed diphtheria/tetanus/pertussis.
Adsorbed diphtheria/tetanus.
Adsorbed diphtheria.
Adsorbed low dose diphtheria vaccine for adults.

Plain vaccines are available but are less immunogenic and have no advantage in terms of reaction rates.

Vaccines should be stored at 2-8° C. The dose is 0.5ml given by intramuscular or deep subcutaneous injection.

5.3 Recommendations

5.3.1 For immunisation of infants and children up to ten years.

a. **Primary immunisation**

Diphtheria vaccine as a component of triple vaccine (diphtheria toxoid, tetanus toxoid and *Bordetella pertussis*) is recommended for infants from two months old. **Adsorbed vaccine should be used as it has been shown to cause fewer reactions than plain vaccine.** If the pertussis component is contraindicated, adsorbed diphtheria/tetanus vaccine should be used. **A course of primary immunisation consists of three doses starting at two months with an interval of one month between each dose** (see 3.6). If a course is interrupted it may be resumed; there is no need to start again.

b. **Reinforcing immunisation**

A booster dose of vaccine containing diphtheria and tetanus toxoids is recommended for children immediately before school entry, preferably after at least three years from the last dose of the primary course.

5.3.2 Immunisation of persons aged ten years or over

a. Primary immunisation

Diphtheria vaccine for adults (**low dose**) MUST be used because of the possibility of a serious reaction in an individual who is already immune. Three doses of 0.5ml should be given by deep subcutaneous or intramuscular injection at intervals of one month.

b. Reinforcing immunisation

A single dose of 0.5ml is required. **This low-dose diphtheria vaccine must be used for all persons aged ten years and over; prior Schick testing is not necessary.**

5.3.3 Children given DTP at monthly intervals without a booster dose at 18 months have been shown to have adequate levels of diphtheria and tetanus antibody at school entry. A booster dose at 18 months for such children is therefore not necessary.

5.3.4 Contacts of a diphtheria case, or carriers.

Individuals exposed to such a risk should be given a complete course or a reinforcing dose according to their age and immunisation history as follows:-

a. **Immunised** children up to ten years.
One injection of diphtheria vaccine.

b. **Immunised** children ten years and over, and adults.
One injection of diphtheria vaccine for adults (low dose).

c. **Unimmunised** children under ten years.
Three injections of diphtheria vaccine at monthly intervals.

d. **Unimmunised** children ten years and over, and adults.
Three injections of diphtheria vaccine for adults (low dose) at monthly intervals.

Unimmunised contacts of a case of diphtheria should in addition be

Immunisation against Infectious Disease

given a prophylactic course of erythromycin.

5.3.5 HIV-positive individuals **may** be immunised against diphtheria in the absence of any contraindications (5.7).

5.4 Use of the Schick test

5.4.1 The Schick test is recommended for individuals who may be exposed to diphtheria in the course of their work. In such cases immunity to diphtheria should be ensured by means of a Schick test carried out at least three months after immunisation is completed.

5.5 Schick test

5.5.1 An intradermal injection of 0.2ml of Schick test toxin is given into the flexor surface of the left forearm and 0.2ml of Schick test control (inactivated toxin) material into the corresponding position of the right forearm, using separate syringes and needles. Readings should be made at 24-48 hours and five to seven days. Comparison of the appearances of the two injection sites will reveal responses attributable to immunity and to allergy. Four types of response may occur:

a. **Schick negative** - No visible reaction on either arm. The subject is IMMUNE and need not be immunised or reinforced.

b. **Schick positive** - An erythematous reaction develops at the site of the toxin injection, becoming evident in 24-48 hours and persisting for seven days or more before gradually fading. The control shows no reaction. The subject is NOT IMMUNE and requires to be immunised or reinforced.

c. **Negative-and-pseudo-reaction** - Both injection sites show similar reactions after 48-72 hours, which fade within five to six days. The reactions are due to hypersensitivity to the components of the test materials. The subject is IMMUNE and need NOT be immunised or reinforced.

d. **Positive-and-pseudo-reaction** - (also called combined reaction). Both injection sites show reactions after 48-72 hours but the reaction in the LEFT arm (toxin) is usually larger and more intense than that on the

RIGHT arm. The control response fades considerably by the fifth to seventh day leaving the positive effect clearly evident. Such combined reactors usually have a basal immunity to diphtheria and should NOT be immunised with a further full course of vaccine. Their immunity can successfully be reinforced by a single injection of diphtheria vaccine for adults (low-dose).

5.6 Adverse reactions

5.6.1 Swelling and redness at the injection site are common. Malaise, transient fever and headache may also occur. A small painless nodule may form at the injection site but usually disappears without sequelae. Severe anaphylactic reactions are rare. Neurological reactions have been reported occasionally.

5.6.2 Severe reactions should be reported to the Committee on Safety of Medicines using the yellow card system.

5.7 Contraindications

See Sections 2.2 and 2.2.1 of General Topics.

5.7.1 a. If a child is suffering from any acute illness, immunisation should be postponed until it has fully recovered. Minor infections without fever or systemic upset are not reasons to postpone immunisation.

b. Immunisation should not proceed in children who have had a severe local or general reaction to a preceding dose (see 4.5.1 b).

5.7.2 When there is a need to control an outbreak, diphtheria vaccine may have to be given to individuals suffering from acute febrile illness. **Low-dose diphtheria vaccine for adults MUST be used for persons aged ten years and over.**

5.8 Diphtheria antitoxin

5.8.1 Diphtheria antitoxin is now only used in suspected cases of diphtheria. Tests with a trial dose to exclude hypersensitivity should

Immunisation against Infectious Disease

precede its use. It should be given without waiting for bacteriological confirmation since its action is specific for diphtheria. It may be given intramuscularly or intravenously, the dosage depending on the clinical condition of the patient. It is no longer used for diphtheria prophylaxis because of the risk of provoking a hypersensitivity reaction to the horse serum from which it is derived. Unimmunised contacts of a case of diphtheria should be promptly investigated, kept under surveillance and given antibiotic prophylaxis and vaccine as in 5.3.

5.9 Supplies

5.9.1 Diphtheria vaccines (5.2.2) EXCEPT low-dose diphtheria vaccine for adults are manufactured and supplied by Wellcome Foundation Ltd. (Tel. 0270 583151). ADSORBED VACCINE MUST BE SPECIFIED OR PLAIN VACCINE WILL BE SUPPLIED.

5.9.2 Low-dose diphtheria vaccine for adults is manufactured by Swiss Serum and Vaccine Institute, Berne, and distributed in the UK by Regent Laboratories Limited, Cunard Road, London NW10 6PN (Tel. 081-965 3637).

5.9.3 Schick Test Toxin and Schick Test Control BP. Manufactured and supplied by Wellcome Foundation Ltd. (Tel. 0270 583151).

5.9.4 Diphtheria antitoxin is supplied in vials containing 2000 Iu per ml. Manufactured by the Swiss Serum and Vaccine Institute, Berne, and distributed in the UK by Regent Laboratories Ltd. Cunard Road , London NW10 6PN (Tel. 081-965 3637).

5.10 Bibliography

Immunity of Children to diphtheria, tetanus and poliomyelitis.
Bainton D, Freeman M, Magrath D, Sheffield F W, Smith J G W.
BMJ 1979; (1), 854-857.

Advantages of aluminium hydroxide adsorbed combined diphtheria, tetanus and pertussis vaccines for the immunisation of infants.
Butler N R, Voyce M A, Burland W L, Hilton M L.

BMJ 1959; (1), 663-666.

Susceptibility to diphtheria.
Report of Ad Hoc Working Group.
Lancet 1978; (i), 428-430.

Immunisation of adults against diphtheria.
Sheffield F W, Ironside A G, Abbott J D.
BMJ 1978; (2), 249-250.

Durability of immunity to diphtheria, tetanus and poliomyelitis after a three dose immunisation schedule completed in the first eight months of life.
Jones E A, Johns A, Magrath D I, Melville-Smith M, Sheffield F.
Vaccine 1989: 7; 300-2.

6 Tetanus

6.1 Introduction

6.1.1 Tetanus is an acute disease characterised by muscular rigidity with superimposed agonising contractions. It is induced by the toxin of tetanus bacilli which grow anaerobically at the site of an injury. The incubation period is between four and 21 days, commonly about ten. Tetanus spores are present in soil and may be introduced into the body during injury, often through a puncture wound, but also through burns or trivial, unnoticed wounds. Tetanus neonatorum due to infection of the baby's umbilical stump is an important cause of death in many countries in Asia and Africa, and cases still occur in the European region. World-wide elimination of neonatal tetanus by the year 2000 is one of the World Health Organisation targets. Tetanus is not spread from person to person.

6.1.2 Effective protection against tetanus is provided by active immunisation which was introduced routinely as part of the primary immunisation of infants from the mid 1950's. From 1960-1969 there were approximately 27 annual deaths in England and Wales in which tetanus was implicated. In 1970 it was recommended in the UK that active immunisation should be universal and that in the treatment of wounds, active immunity to tetanus should be initiated and subsequently completed.

6.1.3 In the 1970s around 20 cases of tetanus were notified annually (in E and W), probably about a third of the actual number. From 1974-8 there were 22 deaths attributed to tetanus with a further 21 in which tetanus was identified. From 1983-87 there were 44 notifications, with only two cases in children under 15 years of age, and 14 in persons aged 65 years and over.

See Graph iii Page 37

6.2 Tetanus vaccine

6.2.1 Immunisation protects by stimulating the production of antitoxin which provides immunity against the effects of the toxin. The immunogen is prepared by treating a cell-free preparation of toxin with formaldehyde

Tetanus

Graph 3

Tetanus Notifications (E&W)
Source: OPCS

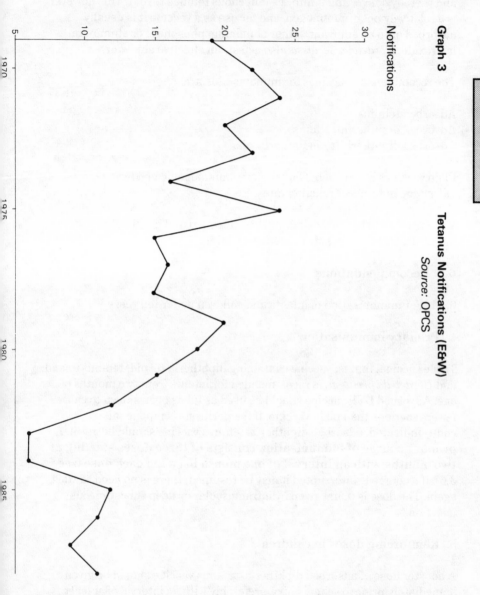

Notifications

Immunisation against Infectious Disease

37

and thereby converting it into the innocuous tetanus toxoid. This however is a relatively poor immunogen, and for use as a vaccine it is usually adsorbed onto an adjuvant, either aluminium phosphate or aluminium hydroxide. *Bordetella pertussis* also acts as an effective adjuvant.

The recommended vaccines for immunisation are:

Adsorbed tetanus.
Adsorbed diphtheria/tetanus.
Adsorbed diphtheria/tetanus/pertussis.

Plain vaccines are available but are less immunogenic and have no advantage in terms of reaction rates.

Vaccines should be stored at 2-8°C. The dose is 0.5ml given by intramuscular or deep subcutaneous injection.

6.3 Recommendations

6.3.1 For immunisation of infants and children under ten years.

a. Primary immunisation

Triple vaccine, that is, vaccine containing diphtheria toxoid, tetanus toxoid, and *Bordetella pertussis*, is recommended for infants from two months of age. Adsorbed DTP vaccine should be used as it has been shown to cause fewer reactions than plain vaccine. If the pertussis component is contraindicated, adsorbed diphtheria/tetanus vaccine should be given. **A primary course of immunisation consists of three doses starting at two months with an interval of one month between each dose** (see 3.6). If a course is interrupted it may be resumed; there is no need to start again. The dose is 0.5ml given by intramuscular or deep subcutaneous injection.

b. Reinforcing doses in children

A booster dose of adsorbed diphtheria/tetanus vaccine should be given immediately prior to school entry, preferably with an interval of at least three years from the last dose of the primary course. If the primary course is only completed at school entry, then the booster dose should be given three years later. A further reinforcing dose of tetanus vaccine alone is recommended for those aged 15-19 years or before leaving school.

6.3.2 Children given DTP at monthly intervals without a booster dose of DT at 18 months have been shown to have adequate antibody levels at school entry. A booster dose at 18 months is therefore not recommended.

6.3.3 For immunisation of adults and children over ten years

a. For primary immunisation, the course consists of three doses of 0.5ml of adsorbed tetanus vaccine by intramuscular or deep subcutaneous injection, with intervals of one month between each dose.

b. A reinforcing dose ten years after the primary course and again ten years later maintains a satisfactory level of protection which will probably be life-long.

c. For immunised adults, booster doses at less than ten year intervals are not recommended since they have been shown to be unnecessary and can cause considerable local reactions.

6.3.4 Treatment of patients with tetanus-prone wounds

The following are considered tetanus-prone wounds:-

a. Any wound or burn sustained more than six hours before surgical treatment.

b. Any wound or burn at any interval after injury that shows one or more of the following characteristics:-

    (i)   A significant degree of devitalised tissue.
    (ii)   Puncture-type wound.
    (iii) Contact with soil or manure likely to harbour tetanus organisms.
    (iv)   Clinical evidence of sepsis.

Thorough surgical toilet of the wound is essential whatever the tetanus immunisation history of the patient.

Specific anti-tetanus treatment is as follows:

Immunisation Status	Type Of Wound Clean	Type Of Wound Tetanus Prone
Last of 3 dose course, or reinforcing dose within last 10 years.	Nil	Nil - (A dose of adsorbed vaccine may be given if risk of infection is considered especially high, eg contamination with stable manure).
Last of 3 dose course or reinforcing dose more than 10 years previously.	A reinforcing dose of adsorbed vaccine.	A reinforcing dose of adsorbed vaccine plus a dose of human tetanus immunoglobulin (6.3.5).
Not immunised or immunisation status not known with certainty.	A full 3 dose course of adsorbed vaccine.	A full 3 dose course of vaccine, plus a dose of tetanus immunoglobulin in a different site.

6.3.5 Specific antitetanus immunoglobulin (see 3.10). See table for recommendations.

Dose

Prevention: 250 Iu, or 500 Iu if more than 24 hours have elapsed since injury, or there is a risk of heavy contamination or following burns.

Treatment: 150 Iu/Kg given in multiple sites.

Available in 1ml ampoules containing 250 Iu.

6.3.6 Routine tetanus immunisation began in 1961, thus individuals born before that year will not have been immunised in infancy. After a tetanus-prone injury such individuals will therefore require a full course of immunisation unless it has previously been given, as for instance in the armed services.

6.3.7 Immunised individuals respond rapidly to a subsequent single injection of adsorbed tetanus vaccine, even after an interval of years.

Immunisation against Infectious Disease

6.3.8 For wounds not in the above categories, such as clean cuts, antitetanus immunoglobulin should NOT be given.

6.3.9 Patients with impaired immunity who suffer a tetanus-prone wound may not respond to vaccine and may therefore require antitetanus immunoglobulin (6.3.5) in addition.

6.3.10 HIV-positive individuals **should** be immunised against tetanus in the absence of contraindications (6.5).

6.4 Adverse reactions

6.4.1 Local reactions, such as pain, redness and swelling around the injection site may occur and persist for several days. General reactions, which are uncommon, include headache, lethargy, malaise, myalgia and pyrexia. Acute anaphylactic reactions and urticaria may occasionally occur and, rarely, peripheral neuropathy. Persistent nodules at the injection site may arise if the injection is not given deeply enough.

6.4.2 Severe reactions should be reported to the Committee on Safety of Medicines using the yellow card system.

6.5 Contraindications

See sections 2.2 and 2.2.1 of General Topics.

6.5.1 a. Tetanus vaccine should not be given to an individual suffering from acute febrile illness except in the presence of a tetanus-prone wound. Minor infections without fever or systemic upset are not reasons to postpone immunisation.

b. Immunisation should not proceed in individuals who have had a severe reaction to a previous dose (see 4.5.1 b.).

6.6 Supplies-vaccine

6.6.1 DTP and DT and T vaccines are manufactured by and available from Wellcome Foundation Ltd. Crewe. (Tel. 0270 583151).

DT Vaccine is also available from:
Evans Medical, Tel.0582 608308

Immunisation against Infectious Disease

Adsorbed tetanus vaccine also available from:
Evans Medical, Tel. 0582 608308.
Merieux UK Ltd. Tel. 0628 785291.
Servier Labs. Ltd, Tel. 02816-2744

6.6.2 Supplies - antitetanus immunoglobulin

Blood Products Laboratory, Tel. 081 953 6191,
Regional Blood Transfusion Centres.
Wellcome (Humotet). Tel. 0270 583151.

6.7 Bibliography

Prevention of tetanus in the wounded.
Smith J W G, Lawrence D R, Evans D G.
BMJ 1975: (iii) 453-455.

Immunity of children to diphtheria, tetanus and poliomyelitis.
Bainton D, Freeman M, Magrath D I, Sheffield F, Smith J W G.
BMJ 1979 (i) 854-857.

Excessive use of tetanus toxoid boosters.
Edsall G, Elliott M W, Peebles T C, Levine L, Eldred M C.
JAMA 1967 202 (i) 17-19.

Duration of immunity after active immunisation against tetanus.
White W G et al.
Lancet 1969 (ii) 95-96.

Reactions after plain and adsorbed tetanus vaccines.
White W G et al.
Lancet 1980 (i) 42.

To give or not to give; guidelines for tetanus vaccine.
Sheffield F W.
Community View (1985) 33, 8-9.

Durability of immunity to diphtheria, tetanus and poliomyelitis after a
three dose schedule completed in the first eight months of life.
Jones E A, Johns A, Magrath D I, Melville-Smith M, Sheffield F.
Vaccine 1989: 7; 300-2.

7 Poliomyelitis

7.1 Introduction

7.1.1 Poliomyelitis is an acute illness following invasion of the gastro-intestinal tract by one of the three types of poliovirus (I, II and III). The virus has a high affinity for nervous tissue and the primary changes are in neurones. The infection may be clinically inapparent, or range in severity from a non-paralytic fever to aseptic meningitis or paralysis. Symptoms include headache, gastro-intestinal disturbance, malaise and stiffness of the neck and back, with or without paralysis. The infection rate in households with young children can reach 100%. The proportion of inapparent to paralytic infections may be as high as 1000 to one in children and 75 to one in adults, depending on the poliovirus type and the social conditions. Poliomyelitis remains endemic in some developing countries where it occurs in epidemics. In countries with an effective immunisation programme the disease occurs as sporadic cases, or in outbreaks amongst unvaccinated individuals. Transmission is through contact with the faeces or pharyngeal secretions of an infected person.

7.1.2 The incubation period ranges from three to 21 days. Cases are most infectious from seven to ten days before and after the onset of symptoms; virus may be shed in the faeces for up to six weeks or longer.

7.1.3 Inactivated poliomyelitis vaccine (Salk) was introduced in 1956 for routine vaccination, and was replaced by attenuated live oral vaccine (Sabin) in 1962. **Individuals born before 1958 may not have been immunised and no opportunity should be missed to immunise them in adult life.** Since the introduction of vaccine,notifications of paralytic poliomyelitis (in E and W) have dropped from nearly 4,000 in 1955 to a total of 35 cases between 1974 -1978. This included 25 cases during 1976 and 1977, in which infection with wild virus occurred in unvaccinated persons, demonstrating the continuing need to maintain high levels of vaccination uptake. From 1986-88, 13 cases were notified; all were either imported or vaccine-associated.

See Graph iv Page 44

Poliomyelitis

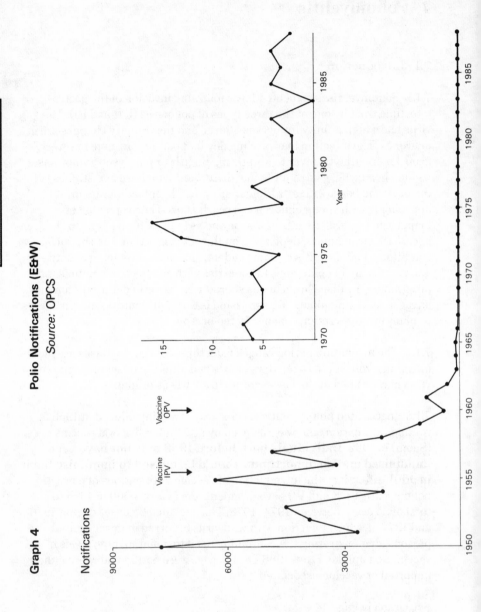

Graph 4

Polio Notifications (E&W)
Source: OPCS

Immunisation against Infectious Disease

7.1.4 By April 1988, 96 of 190 District Health Authorities in England had achieved an uptake of 90% or more for poliomyelitis vaccine.

7.1.5 The World Health Organisation has included the UK among the countries which have eliminated indigenous poliomyelitis.

7.2 Poliomyelitis vaccine (Live and Inactivated)

7.2.1 **Live Oral polio vaccine (OPV)** is routinely used for immunisation in the UK, always given by mouth. It contains live attenuated strains of poliomyelitis virus types I, II and III grown in cultures of monkey kidney cells or on human diploid cells. The attenuated viruses become established in the intestine and promote antibody formation both in the blood and the gut epithelium, providing local resistance to subsequent infection with wild poliomyelitis viruses. This reduces the frequency of symptomless excretion of wild poliomyelitis virus in the community. OPV inhibits simultaneous infection by wild polioviruses and is thus of value in the control of epidemics. Vaccine strain poliomyelitis virus may persist in the faeces for up to six weeks after OPV. Whilst a single dose may give protection, a course of three doses produces long-lasting immunity to all three poliovirus types. OPV should be stored at 0-4°C, and the expiry date should be checked before use. Vaccine stored unopened at 0-4°C is stable, but once the containers are open it may lose its potency. Any vaccine remaining in opened containers at the end of an immunisation session must therefore be discarded.

7.2.2 **Inactivated polio vaccine (IPV)** contains polioviruses of all three types inactivated by formaldehyde. It should be stored at 0-4°C. 0.5ml is given by deep subcutaneous or intramuscular injection (7.3.5). A course of three injections produces long-lasting immunity to all three poliovirus types.

7.3 Recommendations

7.3.1 Primary immunisation of infants and children

Oral poliovaccine is recommended for infants from two months of age. **The primary course consists of three separate doses with intervals of one month between each dose (see 3.6), given at the same time as diphtheria/tetanus/pertussis vaccine.** In infants the dose of three drops

Immunisation against Infectious Disease   45

of vaccine is given from a spoon, whilst in children it can be given on a sugar lump. The dose should be repeated if the vaccine is regurgitated.

7.3.2 Breast-feeding does not interfere with the antibody response to OPV and immunisation should not be delayed on this account.

7.3.3 Faecal excretion of vaccine virus, which can last up to 6 weeks, may lead to infection of unimmunised contacts; usually such infection is of no consequence, but see 2.4.5 and 7.3.9.

7.3.4 The contacts of a recently vaccinated baby should be advised of the need for strict personal hygiene, **particularly for washing their hands after changing the baby's napkins.**

7.3.5 Reinforcing immunisation in children

A reinforcing dose of oral poliomyelitis vaccine (OPV) should be given before school entry at the same time as the reinforcing dose of diphtheria and tetanus vaccine; a further dose of OPV should be given at 15-19 years of age before leaving school.

7.3.6 **Immunisation of adults**

A course of three doses of OPV at intervals of four weeks is recommended for the primary immunisation of adults. **No adult should remain unimmunised against poliomyelitis (see 7.1.3).**

7.3.7 Reinforcing doses for adults are not necessary **unless** they are at special risk, such as:

a. Travellers to areas or countries where poliomyelitis is epidemic or endemic (see "The Traveller's Guide to Health" - T1 1990).

b. Health care workers in possible contact with poliomyelitis cases.

7.3.8 For those exposed to a continuing risk of infection, a single reinforcing dose is desirable every ten years.

7.3.9 Inactivated polio vaccine (IPV) is available for the immunisation of individuals for whom a live vaccine is contraindicated (see 2.2 (iv)). It should also be used for siblings and other household contacts of immuno-suppressed individuals. A primary course of three doses of 0.5ml with intervals of one month should be given by deep subcutaneous or intramuscular injection. Reinforcing doses should be given as for OPV.

7.3.10 HIV-positive asymptomatic individuals **may** receive live polio vaccine but excretion of the vaccine virus in the faeces may continue for longer than in normal individuals. Household contacts should be warned of this and for the need for strict personal hygiene, including hand-washing after nappy changes for an HIV-positive infant.

7.3.11 For HIV-positive symptomatic individuals, IPV may be used instead of OPV at the discretion of the clinician.

7.4 Adverse reactions

7.4.1 Cases of vaccine-associated poliomyelitis have been reported in recipients of OPV and in contacts of recipients. In England and Wales there is an annual average of one recipient and one contact case in relation to over two million doses of oral vaccine. Contact cases would be eliminated if all children and adults were vaccinated. The possibility of a very small risk of poliomyelitis induced by OPV cannot be ignored but is insufficient to warrant a change in vaccination policy. The need for strict personal hygiene for contacts of recent vaccinees must be stressed.

7.4.2 Such cases following immunisation with poliomyelitis vaccine (7.4.1) should be reported to the Committee on Safety of Medicines using the yellow card system.

7.5 Contraindications

See sections 2.2 and 2.2.1 of General Topics.

(i) Febrile illness; immunisation should be postponed.

(ii) Vomiting or diarrhoea.

(iii) Treatment involving high-dose corticosteroids or immunosuppression including general radiation (see 2.2 (iv)).

Immunisation against Infectious Disease

(iv) Malignant conditions of the reticulo-endothelial system such as lymphoma, leukaemia, and Hodgkin's disease, and where the normal immunological mechanism may be impaired as for example, in hypogammaglobulinaemia. See also 2.2 (iv).

(v) Although adverse effects on the fetus have not been reported, oral poliovaccine should not be given to women during the first four months of pregnancy unless there are compelling reasons, such as travel to an endemic poliomyelitis area.

7.5.1 OPV **may** be given at the same time as inactivated vaccines and with other live virus vaccines. If not given simultaneously with other live virus vaccines, an interval of three weeks should be observed. However, when BCG is given to infants, there is no need to delay the primary immunisations which include polio vaccine, because the latter viruses replicate in the intestine to induce local immunity and serum antibodies, and three doses are given.

7.5.2 Both OPV and IPV may contain trace amounts of penicillin and streptomycin but these do not contraindicate their use except in cases of extreme hypersensitivity. Both vaccines contain neomycin in small amounts and OPV may also contain polymyxin.

7.5.3 OPV should NOT be used for the siblings and other household contacts of immunosuppressed children; such contacts should be given IPV.

7.5.4 OPV should be given either three weeks before or three months after an injection of normal immunoglobulin - for instance for hepatitis A (see Section 12). This may not always be possible in the case of travellers abroad, but as in such cases the OPV is likely to be a booster dose the possible inhibiting effect of immunoglobulin is less important.

7.6 Management of outbreaks

7.6.1 After a single case of paralytic poliomyelitis, a dose of OPV should be given to all persons in the immediate neighbourhood of the case (with the exception of individuals with genuine contraindications such as immunodeficiency, 7.5), regardless of a previous history of immunisation

Immunisation against Infectious Disease

against poliomyelitis. **In previously unimmunised individuals the course must be completed.** If there is laboratory confirmation that a vaccine-derived poliovirus is responsible for the case, vaccination of further possible contacts is unnecessary since no outbreaks associated with vaccine virus have been documented to date. If the source of the outbreak is uncertain, it should be assumed to be a "wild" virus and appropriate control measures instituted.

7.7 Supplies

7.7.1 a. Oral poliomyelitis vaccine is available in 10 x 1 dose packs and in dropper tubes of ten doses from:-

Wellcome Foundation (0270 583151).
Smith Kline and French Ltd. (0707 325111).

b. Inactivated poliovaccine (IPV) is supplied in single dose 1ml ampoules. Obtained from;-

Department of Health, 14 Russell Square, WC18 5EP Tel.071-636 6811.
Welsh Health Common Service Authority, Cardiff. Tel. 0222 471234.

7.8 Bibliography

Paralytic poliomyelitis in England and Wales 1976-77.
Collingham K E, Pollock T M, Roebuck M O.
Lancet 1978: (i); 976-977

Effect of breast feeding on sero-response of infants to oral poliovaccine.
John T J, et al.
Pediatrics 1976: 57; 47-53.

Paralytic poliomyelitis in England and Wales 1970-84
Begg N T, Chamberlain R, Roebuck M.
Epidem Inf 1987: 99; 97-106.

Immunity of children to diphtheria, tetanus and poliomyelitis.
Bainton D, Freeman M, Magrath D I et al.
BMJ 1979: (i); 854-857.

Prevalence of antibodies to poliovirus in 1978 among subjects aged 0-88 years.
Roebuck M, Chamberlain R.
BMJ 1982: 284; 697-700.

Prevalence of antibody to poliovirus in England and Wales 1984-86.
White P, Green J.
BMJ 1986: 293; 1153-1155.

Poliomyelitus

8   Measles, Mumps, Rubella

– (for Rubella see also Section 9)

8.1 Introduction

8.1.1 In 1988 combined measles/mumps/rubella (MMR) vaccine was introduced in the UK for young children of both sexes with the aim of eliminating measles, mumps, rubella and the Congenital Rubella Syndrome (CRS). MMR vaccine replaces single antigen measles vaccine; by giving the rubella component to young children it is intended to stop the circulation of rubella and thereby remove the continuing risk of infection to non-immune pregnant women. **Rubella vaccination of girls and non-immune women continues for the foreseeable future (Section 9).**

8.1.2 **Measles** is an acute viral illness transmitted via droplet infection. Clinical features include Koplik spots, coryza, conjunctivitis, bronchitis, rash and fever. The incubation period is about ten days, with a further two to four days before the rash appears. It is highly infectious from the beginning of the prodromal period to four days after the appearance of the rash. Complications have been reported in one in 15 notified cases, and include otitis media, bronchitis, pneumonia, convulsions, and encephalitis, which has an incidence of one in 5000 cases, has a mortality of about 15% and 20 to 40% of survivors have residual neurological sequelae. Electro-encephalographic changes have been reported after apparently uncomplicated measles as well as in cases with frank encephalitis. Complications are more common and severe in poorly nourished and chronically ill children; **it is therefore particularly important that such children should be immunised against measles**.

8.1.3 Notification of measles began in England and Wales in 1940, and until the introduction of vaccine in 1968 annual notifications varied between 160,000 and 800,000, the peaks occurring in two year cycles. By the mid-seventies notifications had fallen to between 50,000 and 180,000. Deaths from measles declined from 1000 in 1940 to 90 in 1968; after the introduction of vaccination the decline continued to an annual average of 13 deaths in the period 1970 to 1988. More than half the deaths occur in previously healthy unvaccinated children. Measles remains a major cause of morbidity and mortality in children receiving immunosuppressive treatment, particularly for leukaemia. Between 1970 and 1983, 19 children

Immunisation against Infectious Disease   51

in remission from acute lymphatic leukaemia died from measles, and of 51 children who died in their first remission in 1974-84, measles was the cause in nearly a third. An additional average of ten deaths a year result from subacute sclerosing panencephalitis, a rare but fatal late complication of measles infection.

See Graph v Page 53

8.1.4 From 1968 to 1980 measles vaccine acceptance for children aged one to two years remained between 50% and 60%. However by April 1989 the overall figure had increased to 80%, with twenty of the 190 English District Health Authorities achieving an uptake of over 90%. Measles notifications in 1989 were the lowest yet recorded.

8.1.5 **Mumps** is an acute viral illness characterised by parotid swelling which may be unilateral or bilateral; some cases are asymptomatic. The incubation period is 14-21 days and mumps is transmissible from several days before the parotid swelling to several days after it appears. Complications include pancreatitis, oophoritis and orchitis; even when the latter is bilateral there is no firm evidence that it causes sterility. Neurological complications including meningitis and encephalitis may precede or follow parotitis, and can also occur in its absence. The trigeminal and facial nerves can be affected by the parotid swelling. Mumps is the cause of about 1200 hospital admissions each year in England and Wales. In the under 15 age group it is a common cause of viral meningitis; it can also cause permanent unilateral deafness at any age.

8.1.6 In the USA where mumps vaccine (as MMR) has been routinely used for over 20 years there has been a dramatic decrease in reported cases of mumps and complications at all ages.

8.1.7 Mumps was made a notifiable disease in the UK in October 1988.

8.1.8 **Rubella** is a mild infectious disease, most common among children aged four to nine years. It causes a transient erythematous rash, lymphadenopathy involving post-auricular and sub-occipital glands and occasionally in adults, arthritis and arthralgia. Clinical diagnosis is unreliable since the symptoms are often fleeting and can be caused by other viruses; in particular, the rash is not diagnostic of rubella. **A history of "rubella" should never be accepted without serological**

Immunisation against Infectious Disease

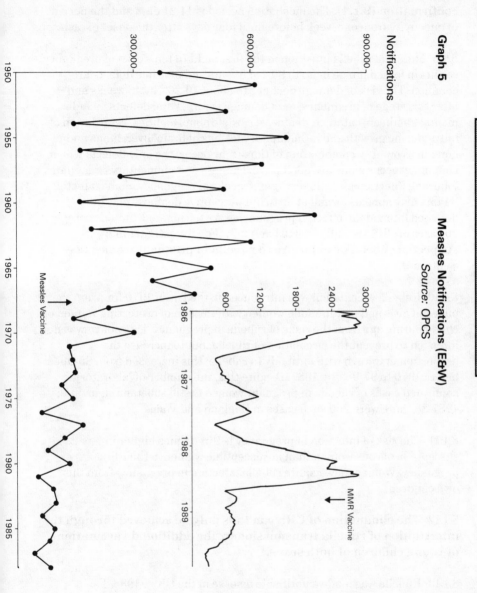

Graph 5

Measles Notifications (E&W)
Source: OPCS

Notifications

900,000

600,000

300,000

1950

1955

1960

1965

1970

1975

1980

1985

Measles Vaccine →

3000
2400
1800
1200
600

1986

1987

1988

1989

MMR Vaccine ←

Measles, Mumps, Rubella

confirmation (9.1.4). The incubation period is 14-21 days and the period of infectivity from one week before until four days after the onset of rash.

8.1.9 Maternal rubella infection in the first eight to ten weeks of pregnancy results in fetal damage in up to 90% of infants and multiple defects are common. The risk of damage declines to about 10-20% by 16 weeks and after this stage of pregnancy, fetal damage is rare. Fetal defects include mental handicap, cataract, deafness, cardiac abnormalities, retardation of intra-uterine growth and inflammatory lesions of brain, liver, lungs and bone-marrow. Any combination of these may occur; the only defects which commonly occur alone are perceptive deafness and pigmentary retinopathy following infection after the first eight weeks of pregnancy. Some infected infants may appear normal at birth but perceptive deafness may be detected later. Many infected pregnancies are terminated, but on average 20 cases of CRS are still reported annually. **For investigation of suspected rubella or exposure to rubella in pregnant women see Section 9**.

8.1.10 Rubella vaccination was introduced in the UK in 1970 for pre-pubertal girls and non-immune women with the aim of protecting women of child-bearing age from the risks of rubella in pregnancy. This policy was not intended to prevent the circulation of rubella, but to increase the proportion of women with antibody to rubella; this increased from 85-90% before 1970 to 97-98% by 1987. Despite this, the number of laboratory-confirmed cases of rubella in pregnant women is still substantial; in 1987-88 there were 260 such cases in England and Wales.

8.1.11 The risk of infection in pregnancy is three times higher in susceptible parous women than in susceptible women in their first pregnancy. Women may acquire rubella infection in pregnancy from their own children.

8.1.12 **The elimination of CRS can thus only be achieved through the interruption of rubella transmission by the additional vaccination of young children of both sexes.**

8.1.13 Rubella was made a notifiable disease in the UK in 1988. For notification of CRS see Section 9.8.

Immunisation against Infectious Disease

8.2 MMR Vaccine

8.2.1 This is a freeze-dried preparation containing live attenuated measles, mumps and rubella viruses. It must be stored in the dry state at 2-8°C (**not frozen**) and protected from light. It should be reconstituted with the diluent supplied by the manufacturer and used within one hour. A single dose of 0.5ml is given by intramuscular or deep subcutaneous injection. Vaccination results in sero-conversion to all three viruses in over 95% of recipients; vaccine-induced antibody to rubella has been shown to persist for at least 16 years in the absence of endemic disease. Since the vaccine viruses are not transmitted, there is **no risk of infection** from vaccinees.

Three vaccines are currently available:-
Pluserix-MMR (Smith Kline and French); Schwartz strain measles, RA27/3 rubella, Urabe Am/9 mumps.

MMR II (Wellcome); further attenuated Enders' Edmonston strain measles, RA 27/3 rubella, Jeryl Lynn mumps.

Immravax (Merieux); Schwartz strain measles, RA 27/3 rubella, Urabe Am/9 mumps.

8.2.2 Single antigen measles, mumps and rubella vaccines are still available. (See Section 9 for Rubella).

8.2.3 **Single antigen rubella vaccine will continue to be given to girls aged 10-14 years and non-immune women before pregnancy and after delivery: see Section 9.**

8.3 Recommendations

8.3.1 MMR vaccine is recommended for children of both sexes aged one to two years unless there is a genuine contraindication (see 8.5). It is also recommended for pre-school children who have not previously received it. **MMR vaccine should be given irrespective of a history of measles, mumps or rubella infection or measles immunisation. There are no ill effects from vaccinating such children**. The target uptake for both these age-groups is at least 90%.

8.3.2 MMR vaccine can be given to children **of any age** whose parents request it, and no opportunity should be missed to ensure that this is done. If the primary course of DTP and polio immunisation has not been completed at the time that MMR vaccine is due, both can be given at the same time using a separate syringe and different sites. Similarly, if children who attend for pre-school immunisation (D/T/polio) have not received MMR vaccine, it should be given then. However since measles, mumps and rubella are most common before the age of entry to secondary school, mass vaccination after the age of 11 when 80-90% have already acquired antibody would currently have little effect on the disease incidence. For maximum effect, vaccine must be given soon after the first birthday, and at the latest before the age of five.

8.3.3 If more than one live virus vaccine needs to be given, they should be given at different sites (unless a combined preparation is used), or at an interval of at least three weeks. If parents do not wish DT and MMR vaccine to be given at the same visit, then OPV should be given with MMR and the child recalled for the DT booster as soon as possible; in these circumstances no three week interval is necessary.

8.3.4 MMR vaccine can be given to non-immune adults and should be considered for those in long-term institutional care who may not have developed immunity.

8.3.5 Children with a personal or close family history of convulsions **should** be given MMR vaccine, provided the parents understand that there may be a febrile response. As for all children, advice for reducing fever should be given (8.4). Doctors should seek specialist paediatric advice rather than refuse vaccination. Dilute immunoglobulin as formerly used with measles vaccine for such children is no longer used since it may inhibit the immune response to the rubella and mumps components.

8.3.6 Unimmunised children in the following groups are at particular risk from measles infection and **should** be vaccinated with MMR vaccine:

a. Children with chronic conditions such as cystic fibrosis, congenital heart or kidney disease, failure to thrive, Down's syndrome.

b. Children from the age of one year upwards in residential or day care including playgroups and nursery schools.

8.3.7 As vaccine-induced **measles** antibody develops more rapidly than that following natural infection, MMR vaccine can be used to protect susceptible contacts during a **measles** outbreak. To be effective the vaccine must be administered within three days of exposure. If there is doubt about a child's immunity, vaccine should be given since there are no ill effects from vaccinating individuals who are already immune. Immunoglobulin is available for individuals for whom vaccine is contraindicated (8.7).

NB. **Antibody response to the rubella and mumps components of MMR vaccine is too slow for effective prophylaxis after exposure to these infections.**

8.3.8 Revaccination is only necessary when vaccine has been given before 12 months of age.

8.3.9 Measles virus inhibits the response to tuberculin, so tuberculin-positive individuals may become tuberculin-negative for up to a month after measles infection or MMR vaccine. Because the measles virus may cause exacerbation of tuberculosis, such patients should be under treatment when immunised.

8.3.10 HIV-positive individuals **may** be given MMR vaccine in the absence of contraindications (8.5).

8.4 Adverse reactions

8.4.1 Malaise, fever and/or a rash may occur, most commonly about a week after vaccination and lasting about two to three days. In a study of over 6000 children aged one to two years the symptoms reported were similar in nature, frequency, time of onset and duration to those commonly reported after measles vaccine. During the sixth to eleventh days after vaccine, febrile convulsions occurred in 1/1000 children, the rate previously reported in the same period after measles vaccine. Parotid swelling occurred in about 1% of children of all ages up to four years, usually in the third week and occasionally later. Culture positive mumps meningo-encephalitis seems to be occuring at a rate of one case per 400,000 distributed doses of vaccine. When mumps virus is isolated from the cerebro-spinal fluid in such cases, laboratory tests can distinguish between wild and vaccine strains. Advice should be sought from the National

8.4.2 Thrombocytopenia, which is usually self-limiting, is occasionally associated with the rubella component, and more rarely, the measles component.

8.4.3 Parents should be told about possible symptoms and given advice for reducing fever, including the use of paracetamol in the period five to ten days after vaccination. They should also be reassured that post-vaccination symptoms are non-infectious.

8.4.4 Serious reactions should be reported to the Committee on Safety of Medicines using the yellow card system.

8.5 Contraindications

See Sections 2.2 and 2.2.1 of General Topics.

(i) Children with acute febrile illness when they present for vaccination; this should be deferred.

(ii) Children with untreated malignant disease or altered immunity; those receiving immunosuppressive or X-ray therapy or high-dose steroids (2.2 (iii), (iv), (v) and 8.7).

(iii) Children who have received another live vaccine – including BCG – within three weeks.

(iv) Children with allergies to neomycin or kanamycin.

(v) If MMR vaccine is given to adult women, pregnancy should be avoided for one month, as for rubella vaccine (9.3.2 and 9.5 (ii)).

(vi) MMR vaccine should not be given within three months of an injection of immunoglobulin.

8.5.1 Allergy to egg

This is only a contraindication if the child has had an anaphylactic reaction (generalised urticaria, swelling of the mouth and throat, difficulty in breathing, hypotension or shock) following food containing egg. Dislike of egg or refusal to eat it is **not** a contraindication. If there is genuine concern, paediatric advice should be sought with a view to vaccination with anti-histamine cover under controlled conditions such as hospital day case admission.

8.6 Supplies

Pluserix-MMR. Smith, Kline and French Tel. 0707 325111.
MMR II. Wellcome Foundation Tel. 0270 583151.
Immravax. Merieux UK Tel. 0628 785291

8.7 Immunoglobulin (and see 3.10)

8.7.1 Measles

Children with compromised immunity (8.5 (ii)) who come into contact with measles should be given human normal immunoglobulin (HNIG) as soon as possible after exposure. Immunocompromised adults without measles antibody should also be given HNIG after exposure to measles.

Children under 12 months in whom there is a particular reason to avoid measles, (such as recent severe illness), can also be given immunoglobulin; MMR vaccine should then be given after an interval of at least three months, at around the usual age.

Dose:

To prevent an attack:

Age	Dose
Under 1 year	250mg
1-2 years	500mg
3 and over	750mg

To allow an attenuated attack:

Under 1 year	100mg
1 year or over	250mg

An interval of at least three months must be allowed before subsequent MMR vaccination.

Immunisation against Infectious Disease 59

Dilute immunoglobulin as previously used with measles vaccine for children with a history of convulsions is no longer used since it may inhibit the immune response to rubella and mumps.

8.7.2 Mumps

HNIG is no longer used for post-exposure protection since there is no evidence that it is effective. Mumps-specific immunoglobulin is no longer available.

8.7.3 Rubella

Post-exposure prophylaxis does **not** prevent infection in non-immune contacts and is therefore **not** recommended for the protection of pregnant women exposed to rubella. It may however reduce the likelihood of clinical symptoms which may possibly reduce the risk to the fetus. It should only be used when termination of pregnancy for proved rubella infection is unacceptable, when it should be given as soon as possible after exposure; serological follow-up of recipients is essential.

Dose: 750mg

8.7.4 Supplies of HNIG:

Central Public Health Laboratory. Tel. 081 200 6868
Public Health Laboratories, England and Wales
Blood Transfusion Service, Scotland
Blood Products Laboratory Tel 081 953 6191.
The Laboratories, Belfast City Hospital Tel. 0232 329241
Immuno, Tel. 0732 458101. (Gammabulin).
Kabivitrum, Tel. 0895 51144 (Kabiglobulin).

Immunisation against Infectious Disease

8.8 Surveillance

The effect of the introduction of MMR vaccine will continue to be assessed by the following methods:-

8.8.1 Uptake of MMR vaccine in each District Health Authority.

8.8.2 Monitoring the proportion of individuals in the population with antibody to measles, mumps and rubella in different age groups.

8.8.3 Monitoring the proportion of ante-natal women susceptible to rubella by age and parity.

8.8.4 Monitoring the number and outcome of rubella infections in pregnancy, terminations for rubella and notified cases of CRS (Section 9).

8.9 Bibliography

Severity of notified measles.
Miller C L.
BMJ 1978; i: 1253

Death from measles.
Miller C L.
BMJ 1985; 290: 443-444.

Mortality and morbidity caused by measles in children with malignant disease attending four major treatment centres: a retrospective view.
Gray M, Hann I M, Glass S, Eden O B, Morris Jones P, Stevens R F.

Measles serology in children with a history of measles in early life.
Adjaye N, Azad A, Foster M, Marshall W C, Dunn H.
BMJ 1983; 286: 1478.

Live measles vaccine: a 21 year follow up.
Miller C L.
BMJ 1987; 295: 22-24.

Safe administration of mumps/measles/rubella vaccine in egg allergic children.

Measles, Mumps, Rubella

Greenberg M A, Birx D L.
J. Pediatrics 1988; 113: 504-6.

Safe immunistion of allergic children against measles, mumps and rubella.
Juntenen-Backman K, Peltola H, Backman A, Salo O P.
Am. J. Dis. Children 1987; 141: 1103-5

Virus meningitis and encephalitis in 1979.
Noah N D, Urquart A M.
J. Infection 1980; 2: 379-83.

Big bang for immunisation. Editorial.
Sir John Badenoch.
BMJ 1988; 297: 750-1.

Surveillance of antibody to measles, mumps and rubella by age.
Morgan-Capner P, Wright J, Miller C, L, Miller E.
BMJ 1988; 297: 770-2

Surveillance of symptoms following MMR vaccine in children.
Miller C L et al.
Practitioner 1989; 233: 69-73.

Mumps meningitis and MMR vaccination.
Lancet 1989, ii: 1015-1016.

Mumps viruses and mumps, measles, and rubella vaccine.
Forsey T, Minor P D.
BMJ 1989; 299: 1340.

For rubella references see Section 9.

9   Rubella

9.1   Introduction

9.1.1   Rubella is a mild infectious disease, most common among children aged four to nine years. It causes a transient erythematous rash, lymphadenopathy involving post-auricular and sub-occipital glands and occasionally in adults, arthritis and arthralgia. Clinical diagnosis is unreliable since the symptoms are often fleeting and can be caused by other viruses; in particular the rash is not diagnostic of rubella. **A history of rubella should therefore not be accepted without serological evidence of previous infection.** The incubation period is 14-21 days, and the period of infectivity is from one week before until four days after the onset of rash.

9.1.2   Maternal rubella infection in the first eight to ten weeks of pregnancy results in fetal damage in up to 90% of infants and multiple defects are common; the Congenital Rubella Syndrome (CRS). The risk of damage declines to about 10-20% by 16 weeks; after this stage of pregnancy fetal damage is rare. Fetal defects include mental handicap, cataract, deafness, cardiac abnormalities, retardation of intra-uterine growth, and inflammatory lesions of brain, liver, lungs and bone-marrow. Any combination of these defects may occur; the only defects which commonly occur alone are perceptive deafness and pigmentary retinopathy following infection after the first eight weeks of pregnancy. Some infected infants may appear normal at birth but perceptive deafness may be detected later. Many infected pregnancies are terminated but on average 20 cases of CRS are reported annually.

9.1.3   Rubella was made a notifiable disease in the UK in 1988. For notification of cases of CRS see 9.8.

9.1.4   **Confirmation of rubella infection in pregnant women**

Because the rash is not diagnostic and also because infection can occur with no clinical symptoms, acute rubella can only be confirmed by laboratory tests. Diagnosis of acute infection requires one of the following:-

a. Paired sera, the first taken within two to three days of onset of rash and the second from eight to nine days after the onset to demonstrate appearance of rubella antibody:

OR

b. A single blood sample from seven days after the onset of rash for estimation of rubella-specific IgM antibody; this may be detectable up to six weeks.

9.1.5 Investigation of pregnant women exposed to rubella

As soon as possible after the exposure to rubella, a blood sample should be taken and sent to the laboratory with **date of LMP and date of exposure.** A second sample should be taken two weeks later and if this is negative, a third sample may be requested after another two weeks.

All pregnant women with suspected rubella or exposed to rubella must be investigated serologically, irrespective of a history of vaccination, clinical rubella or a previous positive rubella antibody result. Close collaboration between virologists and clinicians is essential for the accurate interpretation of serological results and subsequent actions.

9.2 Rubella vaccine

9.2.1 The rubella virus was isolated in cell cultures in 1962. Vaccines are prepared from strains of attenuated virus and have been licensed in the UK since 1970. All rubella vaccine used in the UK contains the Wistar RA 27/3 strain grown in human diploid cells.

9.2.2 Rubella vaccine is a freeze dried preparation. It must be stored in the dried state at 2-8° C (**not** frozen) and reconstituted with the diluent fluid supplied by the manufacturer; it must be used within one hour of reconstitution. For both children and adults the dose is 0.5ml given by deep subcutaneous injection.

9.2.3 One dose of vaccine produces an antibody response in over 95% of vaccinees. In girls who were among the first to be vaccinated in the UK, vaccine-induced antibody has shown little decline after nearly 20 years. In countries where rubella is no longer endemic, vaccine-induced antibody has been shown to persist for at least 16 years. Protection against clinical rubella appears to be long-term even in the presence of declining antibody.

9.2.4 A few recipients fail to produce antibody following vaccination. In addition, a very small number of individuals lose antibody, whether this is derived from natural infection or vaccine. **Women should therefore be screened for rubella antibody in every pregnancy, and at their request, when pregnancy is contemplated. Documented evidence of vaccination must not be accepted as evidence of immunity.**

9.2.5 Rubella infection can occur (but very rarely) in individuals with both natural and vaccine-induced antibody. Occasional cases of CRS after reinfection in pregnancy have been reported; although the risk to the fetus cannot be quantified it is considered to be very low.

9.2.6 Susceptible pregnant women will continue to be at risk of rubella infection in pregnancy until the transmission of rubella virus is interrupted by a sufficiently high uptake of MMR vaccine in young children of both sexes (see Section 8).

9.2.7 The vaccine virus is not transmitted from vaccinees to susceptible contacts. There is thus no risk to pregnant women from contact with recently vaccinated individuals.

9.3 Recommendations (and see Section 8)

9.3.1 a. All girls between their 10th and 14th birthdays should be vaccinated with single antigen rubella vaccine unless there is documented evidence that they have received MMR vaccine already. A history of rubella should be disregarded because of the unreliability of diagnosis. Boys will not be vaccinated at this age because of reasons given in 8.3.1.

This programme will continue with the present target of 95% in order to maintain the current high proportion of women with rubella antibody. Only when there is evidence that a high uptake of MMR vaccine (Section 8) in young children has been achieved

Rubella

and maintained will stopping the schoolgirl rubella programme be considered.

b. Non-pregnant seronegative women of child-bearing age should be given single antigen rubella vaccine and advised not to become pregnant within one month of vaccination. Immigrants who have entered the UK after the age of school vaccination are particularly likely to require vaccination.

9.3.2 Vaccination should be avoided in early pregnancy; doctors should ascertain the date of the LMP before vaccinating. However despite active surveillance in USA, UK and Germany no case of Congenital Rubella Syndrome has been reported following inadvertent vaccination shortly before or during pregnancy (but see 9.8.1). There is thus no evidence that the vaccine is teratogenic; termination of pregnancy following vaccination should therefore **not** normally be routinely recommended. The potential parents should be given this information before making a decision about termination.

9.3.3 General practitioners are uniquely placed to ensure that all women of child-bearing age have been screened for rubella antibody and vaccinated where necessary. Opportunities for screening also arise during ante-natal care, and at family planning, infertility and occupational health clinics. In such cases general practitioners must be informed of the results. Every effort must be made to identify and vaccinate sero-negative women. **All women should be informed of the result of their antibody test** (but see 9.2.4).

9.3.4 Serological testing of non-pregnant women should be performed whenever possible before vaccination, but need not be undertaken where this might interfere with the acceptance or delivery of vaccine. Pregnancy should be avoided for one month.

9.3.5 Women found to be seronegative on ante-natal screening should be vaccinated after delivery and before discharge from the maternity unit. If anti-D immunoglobulin is required, the two may be given at the same time in different sites with separate syringes. While it has now been established that anti-D immunoglobulin does not interfere with the antibody response to vaccine, blood transfusion does inhibit the response in up to 50% of vaccinees. In such cases a test for antibody should be performed eight weeks later, with revaccination if necessary. If rubella vaccine is not given post-partum before discharge, the general practitioner MUST be informed of the need for this. Alternatively it can be given at the post-natal visit. The risk of rubella infection in pregnancy is greater for parous than for nulliparous women because their own children are a source of infection. **All women found on ante-natal screening to be susceptible to rubella should be vaccinated after delivery and before the next pregnancy.**

9.3.6 To avoid the risk of transmitting rubella to pregnant patients, **all health service staff, both male and female,** should be screened and those seronegative vaccinated.

9.3.7 Rubella vaccine **may** be given to HIV positive individuals in the absence of contraindications (9.5).

9.4 Adverse reactions

9.4.1 Mild reactions such as fever, sore throat, lymphadenopathy, rash, arthralgia and arthritis may occur following vaccination. Symptoms usually begin one to three weeks after vaccination and are transient; joint symptoms are more common in women than in young girls. Thrombocytopenia, usually self-limiting, has occasionally been reported after rubella vaccine. Very rarely neurological symptoms have been reported but a causal relationship has not been established.

9.4.2 Serious reactions following rubella vaccination should be reported to the Committee on Safety of Medicines using the yellow card system.

9.5 Contraindications

See Sections 2.2 and 2.2.1 of General Topics.

(i) Rubella vaccine should not be given to a woman known to be pregnant, and pregnancy should be avoided for one month after vaccination, but see 8.3.2.

(ii) Vaccination should be postponed if the patient is suffering from a

Immunisation against Infectious Disease   67

febrile illness until recovery is complete.

(iii) The vaccine should not be administered to patients receiving high dose corticosteroid (see 2.2 (iv)) or immunosuppressive treatment including general radiation; or to those suffering from malignant conditions of the reticulo-endothelial system such as lymphoma, leukaemia, Hodgkin's disease or where the normal immunological mechanism may be impaired as, for example, in hypogammaglobulinaemia.

(iv) If it is necessary to administer more than one live virus vaccine at the same time, these may be given simultaneously at different sites unless a combined preparation is used. If not given simultaneously they should be separated by an interval of at least three weeks. A three week interval should be allowed between the administration of rubella vaccine and BCG.

(v) Rubella vaccine should not be given within three months of an injection of immunoglobulin.

9.5.1 Rubella vaccines contain traces of neomycin and/or polymyxin. Previous anaphylactic reaction to these substances contraindicate rubella immunisation.

9.6 Supplies

Four freeze-dried live vaccines are available, all containing the same strain, Wistar RA 27/3:

Almevax   Wellcome Foundation. Tel. 0270 583151.
Ervevax   Smith Kline and French. Tel. 0707 325111.
Meruvax   Morson. Tel. 0992 467272.
Rubevax   Merieux UK Ltd. Tel. 0628 785291.

9.7 Human normal immunoglobulin (HNIG)

Post-exposure prophylaxis with immunoglobulin does **not** prevent infection in non-immune contacts and is therefore **not** recommended for protection

of pregnant women exposed to rubella. It may however reduce the likelihood of clinical symptoms which may possibly reduce the risk to the fetus. It should only be used if termination for confirmed rubella would be unacceptable when it should be given soon after exposure; serological follow-up of recipients is essential.
Dose: 750mg.
For supplies see 8.7.

9.8 Surveillance of CRS and rubella vaccination in pregnancy

9.8.1 Congenital Rubella Syndrome has been included amongst the rare diseases monitored by the British Paediatric Surveillance Unit which sends monthly enquiries to paediatricians.

9.8.2 Any child with congenital rubella defects, or with symptoms suggestive of congenital rubella, or with laboratory evidence of intra-uterine infection without symptoms should also be notified to the National Congenital Rubella Surveillance Scheme:

Dr. Helen Holzel
Department of Microbiology
Hospital for Sick Children
Great Ormond Street
London WCIN 3JN
Tel. 01-405 9200 ext. 5285/6, 2417

This Department is also investigating the effects of rubella vaccination in pregnancy. If a woman is given rubella vaccine in pregnancy, or becomes pregnant within one month of vaccination, the Department should be notified as soon as possible. Arrangements will then be made for the appropriate clinical and virological examination of the new-born infant, and for subsequent follow-up.

9.9 Bibliography

Consequences of confirmed maternal rubella at different stages of pregnancy.
Miller E, Cradock-Watson J E, Pollock T M.
Lancet 1982; ii: 781-4.
Rubella vaccination: persistence of antibodies for up to 16 years.
O'Shea S, et al.
BMJ 1982; 285: 253.

Rubella antibody persistence after immunisation.
Chu S Y, Bernier R H, Stewart J A et al.
JAMA 1988; 259: 3133-6.

Rubella vaccination and pregnancy: preliminary report of a national survey.
Shepherd S, Smithells R W, Dickson A, Holzel H.
BMJ 1986; 292: 727.

National Congenital Rubella Surveillance Programme 1.7.71-30.6.84.
Smithells R W, Sheppard S, Holzel H, Dickson A.
BMJ 1985: 291; 40-41.

Rational strategy for rubella vaccination.
Hinman A, Orenstein W, Bart K, Preblud S.
Lancet 1983: i; 39-41.

Some current issues relating to rubella vaccine.
Preblud S.
JAMA 1985; 254 (2): 253-6.

Effect of selective vaccination on rubella susceptibility and infection in pregnancy.
Miller C L, Miller E, Sequeira P J, Cradock-Watson J E, Longson M, Wiseberg E.
BMJ 1985; 291: 1398-1401.

Rubella

Immunisation against Infectious Disease

Rubella susceptibility and the continuing risk of infection in pregnancy.
Miller C L, Miller E, Waight P A.
BMJ 1987; 294: 1277-8.

Congenital rubella in babies of south Asian women in England and Wales: an excess and its causes.
Miller E, Nicoll A, Rousseau S, Sequeira P J L, Hambling M H, Smithells RW, Holzel H.
BMJ 1987; 294: 737-739.

Outcome of periconceptional maternal rubella.
Enders G, Nickerl-Packer U, Miller E, Cradock-Watson J E.
Lancet 1988; 11: 1445-6.

Rubella

10 Tuberculosis: BCG Vaccination

10.1 Introduction

10.1.1 Human tuberculosis is caused by infection with *Mycobacterium tuberculosis* or *Mycobacterium bovis* which may affect any part of the body. In the UK, 90% of new cases involve the respiratory system but non-respiratory forms are more common in immigrant ethnic groups and when past infection is reactivated (especially in those who are immunocompromised). The infection is now most commonly acquired by aerosol spread and such transmission is most likely when the index case is sputum smear-positive for the bacillus.

10.1.2 In the UK, the incidence of the disease has declined tenfold since 1948 (see Graph) but high immigration levels in the late 1960s (particularly from the Indian subcontinent) materially slowed the decline. The incidence is higher in Scotland and it varies widely in England and Wales partly as a consequence of this immigration. During 1988 in England and Wales there were 5,161 new cases notified and 718 deaths. Although case fatalities decreased rapidly with the introduction of effective chemotherapy forty years ago, the ratio of deaths to new cases has never fallen below 9.9% and was 13.9% in 1988.

See Graph vi Page 73

10.1.3 After initial trials in the UK, the more general use of BCG vaccine started in 1953. National coverage at age 13 by comprehensive school programmes was incomplete for many years but had reached 35% of the target age-cohort in 1958 and 60% by 1962. In the last decade it has averaged 75% of the target group of which a further 7% are tuberculin positive. The protective efficacy of the vaccine is high and BCG vaccination is particularly important for those at high-risk of infection, for immigrants from high-prevalence areas, and for those intending to stay in such areas.

10.2 Bacillus Calmette-Guerin vaccine (intradermal)

10.2.1 BCG vaccine (intradermal) contains a live attenuated strain derived

Immunisation against Infectious Disease

Graph 6

Tuberculosis Notifications (E&W)

Source: OPCS

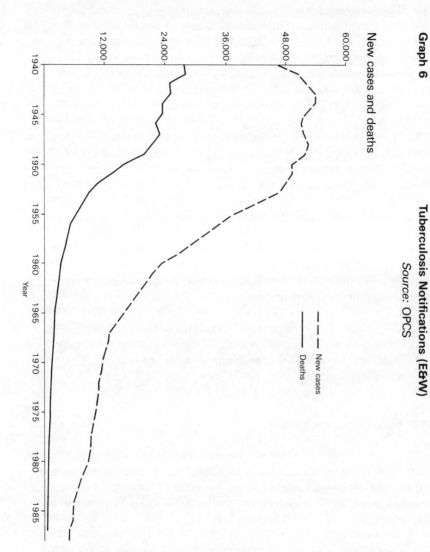

New cases and deaths

- - - New cases

—— Deaths

from *Mycobacterium bovis.* It is now available freeze-dried in rubber-capped vials with diluent in a separate ampoule. It is supplied to NHS users without charge by District Health Authorities who order it from the appropriate government Health Department (see section 10.10). This vaccine has been shown to protect against tuberculosis with efficacy greater than 70% in British schoolchildren. Protection lasts at least 15 years with little attrition of effectiveness.

10.2.2 The freeze-dried BCG vaccine (as supplied and before reconstitution) should be protected from light, stored between 2° and 8°C, and never frozen. It has a shelf life of 12 months and should not be used after the expiry date stated on the label.

10.2.3 The multidose vial of vaccine should be diluted as instructed on the package insert using aseptic precautions, a syringe and suitable large needle. The needle may be left *in situ* for subsequent withdrawal of vaccine. Following reconstitution, the vaccine should be used in one session or discarded. Reconstituted vaccine should never be kept longer than the end of the session in which it is prepared.

10.2.4 For tuberculosis contacts on isoniazid prophylactic therapy, isoniazid-resistant BCG vaccine is available and should be ordered by the user direct from the manufacturer Evans Medical Ltd or through a pharmaceutical wholesaler.

10.3 Vaccination technique

10.3.1 It is recommended that BCG vaccine be administered intradermally using a tuberculin syringe and needle. **Jet injectors should not be used and the percutaneous route (using a modified Heaf gun) is also not recommended.** BCG vaccine should not be given within three weeks of any other live vaccine whichever is given first.

10.3.2 For all vaccinees except newly-born babies, a tuberculin skin test must be carried out first so that BCG is **never** administered to those who show a positive reaction to tuberculoprotein. The approved techniques of tuberculin skin testing are described in section 10.7.

10.3.3 The dose of BCG vaccine is 0.1ml for all ages except infants under three months when it is reduced to 0.05ml. It is injected intradermally using a syringe and needle. The needle should be 0.5 x 10mm (25 gauge about 3/8″ long) and have a short bevel. The use of a separate **syringe and needle** for each patient is essential to avoid the risk of transmission of hepatitis, HIV etc.

10.3.4 Careful identification of the site of inoculation is important and this should be at the **insertion of the deltoid muscle onto the humerus** (see Figure) which is not much higher than the middle of the upper arm. Sites higher on the arm are more likely to lead to keloid formation, the tip of the shoulder most of all. In girls, for cosmetic reasons, the upper and lateral surface of the thigh may be preferred.

See fig.1 page 76

10.3.5 Before the intradermal injection, the skin should be swabbed with spirit and allowed to dry. The operator should stretch the skin between the thumb and forefinger of one hand and with the other slowly insert the needle, with the bevel upwards, for about 2mm into the superficial layers of the dermis almost parallel with the surface. The correct needle (see paragraph 10.3.3.) has a short bevel which can usually be seen through the epidermis during insertion (these needles should not be used to penetrate the rubber cap of the vial).

10.3.6 A raised blanched bleb showing the tips of the hair follicles *(peau d'orange)* is a sign that the injection has been made correctly and a bleb typically of 7mm diameter follows 0.1ml injection.

10.3.7 The injection must be given intradermally and particular care should be taken to avoid accidental subcutaneous injection **of any part of the dose.** Considerable resistance is felt when correctly giving an intradermal injection. If this resistance is not felt and it is suspected that the needle may be too deep, it should be removed and reinserted elsewhere before more vaccine is given.

10.3.8 **Vaccination reaction**

Normally a local reaction develops at the site of the vaccination within two to six weeks, beginning as a small papule which increases in size for a few weeks. Occasionally a shallow ulcer up to 10mm in diameter may develop. If

Figure 1
Injection site and technique

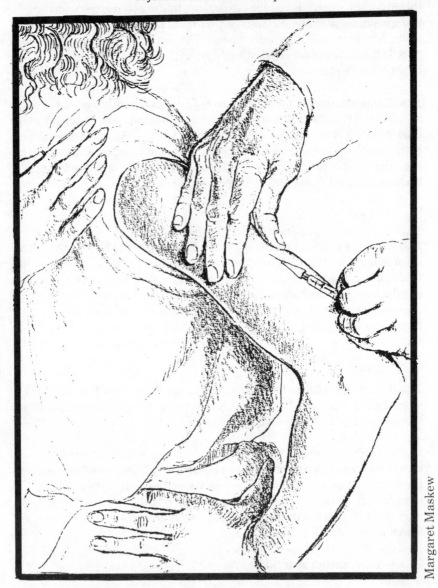

Margaret Maskew

Figure

The technique of administering BCG vaccine by intradermal injection into the upper arm at the site of the insertion of the deltoid muscle onto the humerus.

Tuberculosis: BCG Vaccination

this discharges, a temporary dry dressing may be used until a scab forms, but it is essential that air should not be excluded.

10.3.9 If absolutely essential, an impermeable dressing may be applied but only for a short period (for example, to permit swimming) as it may delay healing and cause a larger scar. The lesion slowly subsides over several months and eventually heals leaving only a small scar.

10.3.10 After inoculation with BCG vaccine there is a high tuberculin conversion rate and further observation of those at **normal risk** is not necessary, nor is further tuberculin testing recommended. However, in large vaccination programmes, a check should be made for adverse reactions six weeks or so later, possibly on a sample basis.

10.3.11 After vaccination of those at **higher risk,** subsequent inspection of the site is a matter for clinical discretion. However, when vaccine is administered to **health-care staff judged to be at high risk**, the site of vaccination should be inspected six weeks later to confirm that a satisfactory reaction has occurred. Those who show no reaction to BCG require a post-BCG, tuberculin test, after which anyone who is still tuberculin negative should be re-vaccinated (see paragraph 10.4.4. *et seq*).

10.4 Recommendations

10.4.1 It is recommended that the following groups be vaccinated with BCG provided:

    a. Previous **successful** BCG vaccination has not been carried out.

    b. The tuberculin skin test is negative (as defined in paragraph 10.7.14 *et seq*).

Past successful BCG vaccination will have produced a characteristic scar (usually on the upper arm or lateral aspect of the thigh) which may be supported by a history of vaccination. Newly-born babies may be vaccinated without prior skin testing. Revaccination with BCG is only advised for those at higher risk who failed to develop a reaction and scar following earlier vaccination (and are tuberculin negative).

Immunisation against Infectious Disease

10.4.2 Those at **normal risk:**

    a. School children between the ages of 10 and 13 years.
    b. All students including those in teacher training colleges.
    c. Newly-born babies, children or adults where the parents or the
individuals request BCG vaccination.

10.4.3 Those at **higher risk:**

    a. Health service staff considered to be at high risk from contact with
infectious patients or their specimens. These comprise doctors, nurses,
physiotherapists, radiographers, occupational therapists, technical staff
in microbiology and pathology departments including attendants in
autopsy rooms, students in all these disciplines, and any others
considered to be at high risk. It is particularly important to test and
vaccinate staff working in maternity and paediatric departments.
    b. Veterinary and other staff who handle animal species known to be
susceptible to tuberculosis eg simians.
    c. Contacts of cases known to be suffering from active respiratory
tuberculosis. Newly-born babies who are contacts should be vaccinated
immediately.
    d. Immigrants from countries with a high prevalence of tuberculosis,
their children and infants wherever born. Vaccination of these babies is
recommended within a few days of birth.
    e. Those intending to stay in Asia, Africa, Central or South America for
more than a month.

10.4.4 **Health-care staff at high risk**

Health-care staff are at high risk if they are in contact with tuberculous
patients or tuberculous pathological material. They need further
observation following BCG vaccination. Staff in this high risk group should
have the site of vaccination inspected six weeks after inoculation to confirm
that a satisfactory reaction has occurred. Only those who show no evidence
of a reaction require a post-BCG tuberculin test, after which anyone who is
tuberculin negative should be re-vaccinated.

10.4.5 If after revaccination there is still no evidence of a satisfactory
reaction or of conversion to a positive tuberculin test, the subject should be
moved to work of lower risk where he will not be exposed to patients with

tuberculosis or to tuberculous material.

10.4.6 Post-vaccination tuberculin tests should be carried out 6 to 12 weeks after vaccination. In the meantime, staff who have failed to show a satisfactory local response to vaccination should be excluded from high risk activity.

10.4.7 Contacts of tuberculosis.

Vaccination will do no harm if performed in a subject with recently acquired tuberculosis infection (where the skin test was negative because tuberculin sensitivity had not developed). However, there is advantage in delaying BCG vaccination for about six weeks if the contact proves to be tuberculin negative on the first test after segregation of a sputum smear-positive index case.

10.4.8 Six weeks after segregation of the index case, the skin test on the contact should be repeated and vaccination carried out only if this test is negative. It is however better to vaccinate without segregation than not to vaccinate at all.

10.4.9 Prophylactic isoniazid may be administered to a contact and isoniazid-resistant BCG vaccine should than be used for vaccination (see paragraph 10.2.4).

10.4.10 Immigrants

New entrants to the UK from countries where tuberculosis is of high prevalence (eg the Indian subcontinent) must be tuberculin skin-tested as part of the initial screening procedure. Those with strongly positive reactions (see paragraph 10.7.14 *et seq*) may require chemotherapy or further follow-up at a chest clinic. BCG vaccination should be offered immediately to those who are tuberculin negative, and their infants born subsequently in this country should be vaccinated soon after birth.

10.4.11 Infants and babies

Where BCG vaccination of infants is recommended, it may be carried out soon after birth and newly-born babies, even if contacts, need not be tested for tuberculin sensitivity beforehand. Otherwise infants may be vaccinated at any age following skin-testing, although BCG must not be administered within three weeks of any other live vaccine (see paragraph 10.6.2). The dose of BCG is reduced to 0.05ml for infants under three months. As for adults, a separate syringe and needle must be used for each infant. **Jet injectors should not be used.**

10.5 Adverse reactions to BCG vaccine

10.5.1 Severe injection site reactions, large ulcers and abscesses are most commonly caused by faulty injection technique where part or all of the dose is administered too deeply (subcutaneously instead of intradermally). The vaccination of individuals who are tuberculin positive may also give rise to such reactions. To avoid these, doctors and nurses who carry out tuberculin skin tests and administer BCG vaccine must be trained in the interpretation of the results of tuberculin tests as well as in the technique of intradermal injection with syringe and needle.

10.5.2 Keloid formation at the injection site is a not uncommon but largely avoidable complication of BCG vaccination. Some sites are more prone to keloid formation than others and vaccinators should adhere to the two sites recommended in this chapter (the mid-upper arm or the thigh). Most experience has been gained in the use of the upper arm and it is known that the risk of keloid formation is increased manyfold when the injection is given at a site higher than the **insertion of the deltoid muscle onto the humerus** (see paragraph 10.3.4).

10.5.3 Apart from these injection site reactions, other complications following BCG vaccination are rare and mostly consist of adenitis with or without suppuration and discharge. A minor degree of adenitis may occur in the weeks following vaccination and should not be regarded as a complication. Very rarely a lupoid type of local lesion has been reported. A few cases of widespread dissemination of the injected organisms have been reported and anaphylactic reactions can occur.

10.5.4 It is important that all complications should be recorded and reported to a chest physician. Serious or unusual complications (including abscess and keloid scarring) should be reported to the Committee on Safety of Medicines using the yellow card system. Every effort should be made to recover and identify the causative organism from any lesion constituting a serious complication.

Immunisation against Infectious Disease

10.6 Contraindications

10.6.1 BCG vaccine should NOT be given to subjects:

a. Receiving corticosteroid or other immunosuppressive treatment including general radiation (see paragraph 2.2. (iii), (iv), (v)).

b. Suffering from malignant conditions such as lymphoma, leukaemia, Hodgkin's disease or other tumours of the reticuloendothelial system.

c. Whom the normal immunological mechanism may be impaired, as in hypogammaglobulinaemia.

d. Known to be infected with the AIDS virus (HIV).

e. Who are pregnant (although no harmful effects on the fetus have been observed from BCG vaccination during pregnancy, it is wise to avoid vaccination in the early stages and if possible to delay until after delivery).

f. With positive sensitivity tests to tuberculoprotein (see section 10.7).

g. With pyrexia.

h. With generalised septic skin conditions (but if eczema exists, a vaccination site should be chosen that is free from skin lesions).

10.6.2 An interval of at least three weeks should be allowed between the administration of BCG vaccine and any other live vaccine, whichever is given first. No further immunisation should be given for at least three months in the arm used for BCG vaccination because of the risk of regional lymphadenitis.

10.6.3 However, when BCG is given to infants, there is no need to delay the primary immunisations which include polio vaccine, because the latter viruses replicate in the intestine to induce local immunity and serum antibodies, and three doses are given.

10.7 The tuberculin skin test

10.7.1 Except in newly-born babies, this test should aways be carried out before BCG vaccination and in those where tuberculosis infection is suspected. The test assesses the individual's sensitivity to tuberculoprotein and may provide evidence of past infection or of past successful vaccination. Above all, those who show hypersensitivity to tuberculoprotein may need further investigation and should not be given BCG (but see the definition of positive reactors in paragraph 10.7.14 *et seq*).

10.7.2 Tuberculin testing techniques.

Uniformity of results is essential and a standard recommended technique should be used with the specified preparation of purified protein derivative

(PPD) which users can obtain from their District Health Authority free of charge. Care must be taken to ensure that the dilution of PPD is that specified for the technique to be used. The various preparations of PPD are described in paragraph 10.7.4.

10.7.3 All the common techniques of tuberculin skin testing have been considered for their reliability, ease of use, and safety. Only two methods are recommended for general use: the Mantoux test and the Heaf test. **It is strongly recommended that one of these two techniques be used.** In their application, careful attention should be given to precautions to prevent any risk of cross-infection.

10.7.4 Purified protein derivative (PPD)

Tuberculin Purified Protein Derivative (PPD) BP is a sterile preparation made from the heat-treated products of growth and lysis of the appropriate mycobacterium at a strength of 100,000 units/ml. This strength is however only used for the Heaf test and three dilutions of PPD are available for the Mantoux test. It is very important that the correct strength be used:

Strength units/ml	Dilution of PPD	Units in dose of 0.1ml	Main use
1,000	1 in 100	100	*see note below
100	1 in 1,000	10	Mantoux test (routine)
10	1 in 10,000	1	Mantoux test (special)

*this dilution is only used for special diagnostic purposes

10.7.5 All tuberculin PPD must be stored between 2° and 8°C (never frozen) and protected from light. Once an ampoule is opened, its contents should be used within an hour and not retained beyond the one session. PPD tends to adsorb onto the syringe surface and the injection should therefore be made immediately after it is filled. Note that PPD may persist on the surface of any non-disposable syringe and on the endplate and needles of the Heaf gun, both of which need careful cleaning subsequently.

10.7.6 The Mantoux test

The Mantoux test uses a 1ml syringe and a short bevel 0.5 × 10mm needle (25 gauge about 3/8″ long) as for BCG vaccination itself. A separate

Immunisation against Infectious Disease

syringe and needle must be used for each subject to prevent cross-infection. The test is normally performed on the flexor surface of the forearm but the technique of intradermal injection is the same as that described for BCG vaccination in paragraph 10.3.5 et seq.

10.7.7 An area of skin over the upper third of the flexor surface of the forearm is cleaned with spirit and 0.1ml of tuberculin PPD dilution 100 units/ml is injected intradermaly so that a bleb (*peau d'orange*) is produced typically of 7mm diameter. The results should be read 48 to 72 hours later but usually a valid reading can be obtained up to 96 hours. A positive result consists of induration of at least 5mm diameter following injection of 0.1ml PPD 100 units/ml.

10.7.8 The PPD preparation for routine use in the Mantoux test(dilution 100 units/ml) is supplied in ampoules containing 1.0ml, the contents of an ampoule being sufficient for five or six tests. For tests in patients in whom tuberculosis is suspected, or who are known to be hypersensitive to tuberculin, a dilution of 10 units/ml should be used. This dilution is not supplied routinely through health authorities and should be ordered by users direct from Evans Medical or through a pharmaceutical wholesaler.

10.7.9 **The multiple puncture test (Heaf test)**

For this test the Heaf Multiple Puncture Apparatus (commonly known as Heaf gun) is used with a needle-block of six needles. The puncture depth is adjustable and should be set to 2mm for adults and all children aged two years or more; under that age 1mm is sufficient.

10.7.10 An alternative version of the Heaf gun has a magnetic head that holds a 6-point steel-plate (instead of a needle-block) which is replaced between patients. The steel plate is either discarded or sterilised for re-use. Studies have shown a high false negative rate for this technique and the magnetic head itself may become contaminated with body fluids and require disinfection between patients. It has not proved possible to recommend a method of disinfection for the magnetic head that presents fewer practical difficulties than the method described here for fixed-head guns. **Use of this device is therefore not recommended**.

10.7.11 PPD for the Heaf test contains 100,000 units/ml and is supplied in packs of five ampoules, of 1.0ml, each ampoule normally being sufficient for 20 or more tests depending very much on technique.

10.7.12   A clean dry area of skin on the flexor surface of the forearm is used for this test. If cleaning is necessary, spirit should be used but it is important that the spirit be allowed to evaporate **completely** before the test. The solution of PPD is applied with a sterile glass rod or platinum loop which should not be allowed to come into contact with the skin. The PPD is smoothed over the skin by the end plate of the apparatus, which is then pressed firmly at right angles to the skin surface and the needles released. Excess PPD is then removed. No dressing is needed.

10.7.13   Results may be read any time from 3 to 10 days after puncture. A positive result should be recorded only when there is palpable induration around at least four puncture points. Four grades of response are defined for the Heaf test:-

Grade 1   at least 4 small indurated papules

Grade 2   an indurated ring formed by confluent papules

Grade 3   solid induration 5 to 10mm wide

Grade 4   induration over 10mm wide

10.7.14   **Positive reactors**

It is now generally accepted that a Heaf Grade 1 reaction in an individual who has **not previously received BCG vaccination** does not indicate past infection with *Mycobacterium tuberculosis* or *Mycobacterium bovis*. BCG vaccination may therefore be offered in the absence of contraindications.

10.7.15   Those with reactions of Grade 2 or more are hypersensitive to tuberculoprotein and should not be given BCG vaccine. The equivalent response for the Mantoux test is induration of diameter 5mm or more following injection of 0.1ml PPD 100 units/ml.

10.7.16   The tuberculin reaction in those previously vaccinated with BCG is usually weak and is unlikely to **exceed** Grade 2 (or a Mantoux response with induration of diameter 5 to 14mm after 0.1ml PPD 100 units/ml). A more strongly positive reaction after vaccination may therefore indicate infection prior or subsequent to BCG administration and merits further investigation.

10.7.17 **All** those who show a strongly positive reaction to tuberculin should be referred for further investigation and supervision (which may include prophylactic chemotherapy). A strongly positive reaction is a Heaf response of Grade 3 or 4 or a Mantoux response with induration of at least 15mm diameter following 0.1ml PPD 100 Units/ml.

10.8 Disinfection and maintenance of the Heaf gun

10.8.1 The Heaf gun requires careful maintenance and cleaning between sessions plus replacement or disinfection of the needle-block head **between each subject**. If a sufficient number of spare heads is available, the use of a replacement autoclaved head for each patient is satisfactory. Otherwise the head must be disinfected.

10.8.2 The disinfection technique has been modified after consideration of the risks of virus transmission. The procedure recommended below is virucidal but must be performed carefully. It uses highly flammable spirit and proper precautions are needed to prevent fire hazard.

10.8.3 Disinfection of the Heaf gun should be carried out before each test and at the conclusion of the tuberculin testing session. The recommended method of disinfection is a three-stage process which requires an interval of three minutes or more between consecutive tests with any one instrument. Therefore at least three guns should be available for each team and they should be disinfected and used in rotation. These guns will sustain a testing rate of 60 patients an hour with the required interval for disinfection and cooling.

10.8.4 Only Industrial Methylated Spirit BP should be used. This is a colourless preparation containing 95% ethyl alcohol adulterated with wood naphtha which will burn readily. Note that this is a volatile liquid that may create a highly flammable vapour which should not be left in an open vessel near a naked flame. Mineralised methylated spirits (the violet preparation sold retail for general use) and Surgical Spirit BP contain only 90% alcohol plus other adulterant substances that may inhibit flammability. They are not satisfactory.

10.8.5 The three stages of the disinfection process are immersion in spirit, burning-off of the spirit, and cooling of the gun. The correct application of each stage is essential. For example, immersion to an excessive depth in spirit will cause overheating during burning-off (and possibly a fire risk) which will then require an extended cooling time.

10.8.6 The end of the instrument should first be immersed in the spirit to a depth that totally covers the end-plate and the needles but does not wet the body of the gun. This should be done in a substantial heavy vessel which will support the gun and ensure immersion at the correct depth for at least 2 minutes.

10.8.7 The gun is then withdrawn and held at an angle of 45° to the vertical with the end-plate directed upwards. The spirit is set alight by momentary contact with a flame from which the gun is removed on ignition. The spirit is allowed to burn until the flame goes out. A further 30 seconds should be allowed for cooling, but ensure that the needles do not become contaminated prior to use. **NEVER use a Heaf gun unless you have personally supervised its disinfection in this manner**.

10.8.8 **Maintenance of the Heaf gun**

The Heaf gun should be checked carefully before use to ensure that the needles are sharp, clean and not displaced in their retaining plate. It is good practice to replace needles every six months if the gun is in regular use. Cleaning between tuberculin testing sessions can be carried out using hot detergent solution and a stiff brush, but thorough rinsing in distilled water after cleaning is important. Periodical servicing of the guns by the manufacturer is recommended.

10.9 Record keeping and surveillance

10.9.1 It is important that records be maintained to show the result of tuberculin skin testing and the vaccination state of every person covered by the programme. These records should show who administered the skin test or vaccine and who recorded the result or lesion. Particular attention should be paid to unusual or severe reactions. Such records should be kept for at least ten years.

10.9.2 The results of tuberculin skin tests and of BCG vaccination of

Immunisation against Infectious Disease

hospital staff (including students) should be recorded on appropriate records. If staff or students move to another hospital or to another training school, the record cards should be transferred to the occupational health unit.

10.10 Supplies of BCG vaccine and PPD

10.10.1 In England, supplies of freeze-dried BCG vaccine (intradermal) and Tuberculin PPD are distributed to District Health Authorities once a month. DHAs should make the two products available to users without charge. Orders for at least one month's requirement should be submitted on the DHAs own order form to reach the Department of Health by the first day of the month preceding the month when the materials are required, eg materials for use in August should be ordered by 1st July. The order should be sent to:

> Department of Health
> Procurement Directorate
> 14 Russell Square
> London WC1B 5EP
> 071-636 6811

10.10.2 In Scotland, the Health Boards order BCG vaccine direct from Vestric as and when required but Tuberculin PPD is distributed to users direct every month and should be ordered from:

> The Central Infusion Laboratory
> Knightswood Hospital
> Glasgow G13 2XG
> 041-954 8183

10.10.3 In Wales, orders for both BCG vaccine and PPD should be sent monthly by health authorities (as for England) to:

> Welsh Health Common Services Authority
> Heron House
> 35-43 Newport Road
> Cardiff CF2 1SB
> 0222-471234 extension 2068

10.10.4 In Northern Ireland, Health and Social Services Boards order both BCG vaccine and PPD from:

> Central Services Agency
> 27 Adelaide Street
> Belfast BT2 8FH
> 0232-324431

10.10.5 Those who require isoniazid-resistant BCG vaccine or non-routine strengths of PPD should order direct from:

> Evans Medical Ltd
> Distribution Centre
> Foster Avenue
> Woodside Park Estate
> DUNSTABLE Bedfordshire LU5 5TA
> 0528-608308
> Telefax 0582-600421

10.11 Bibliography

Tuberculosis and human immunodeficiency virus infection.
Chaisson R E and Slutkin G.
J Infect Dis 1989; 159; 96-100.

Tuberculosis and Chest Diseases Unit.
Medical Research Council.

National survey of notifications of tuberculosis in England and Wales in 1983.
BMJ 1985; 291; 658-61.

Tuberculosis among immigrants to England and Wales:
a national survey in 1965.
British Tuberculosis Association.
Tubercle 1966; 47; 145-56

Effectiveness of BCG vaccination in England and Wales in 1983.
Sutherland I and Springett V H.
Tubercle 1987; 68; 81-92

The prevalence of keloid formation in BCG scars.
Lunn J A and Robson D C.
Personal communication.

The Heaf test: a comparison of two types of Heaf gun.
MacHale E M and O'Shea M E B.
Irish Medical Journal 1987; 80; 400-401.

The tuberculin test in clinical practice: an illustrated guide.
Caplin Maxwell.
Bailliere Tindall, London (1980).

11 Influenza

11.1 Introduction

11.1.1 Influenza is an acute viral disease of the respiratory tract characterised by the abrupt onset of fever, chills, headache, myalgia and sometimes prostration. Coryza and sore throat are common and a dry cough is almost invariable. It is usually a self-limiting disease with recovery in two to seven days. There is serological evidence of asymptomatic infection. Influenza is highly infectious, spreading rapidly in institutions. It derives its importance from the speed with which epidemics evolve and the severity of the complications, notably bacterial pneumonia. These features account for the widespread morbidity affecting all age groups, but particularly the elderly and chronic sick. Mortality, measured by the number of excess deaths attributed to "influenza", is in the region of three to four thousand even in winters when the incidence is low.

11.1.2 There are three types of influenza virus: A, B and C, the latter being of little importance. Epidemic influenza is usually caused by influenza A which attacks all age-groups, with the highest incidence in children and adolescents. Outbreaks due to Influenza A occur in most years, those due to Influenza B at intervals of several years. Influenza A viruses are antigenically labile and the principal surface antigens, the haemagglutin and neuraminidase, undergo antigenic changes. Major changes (so-called 'antigenic shifts') occur periodically and are responsible for the emergence of sub-types which may cause pandemics. More minor changes (so-called 'antigenic drifts') occur more frequently and are responsible for the interpandemic prevalence of influenza. Marked antigenic drift may be followed by large winter epidemics, but it is rarely possible to forecast the extent of outbreaks.

See Graph vii Page 91

11.2 Influenza vaccine

11.2.1 Influenza vaccine formulation is reviewed annually and when significant alterations in antigen have occurred; changes in the composition are made to counter these 'antigenic shifts' and 'antigenic drifts'.

Graph 7

Incidence of Influenza
Source: RCGP

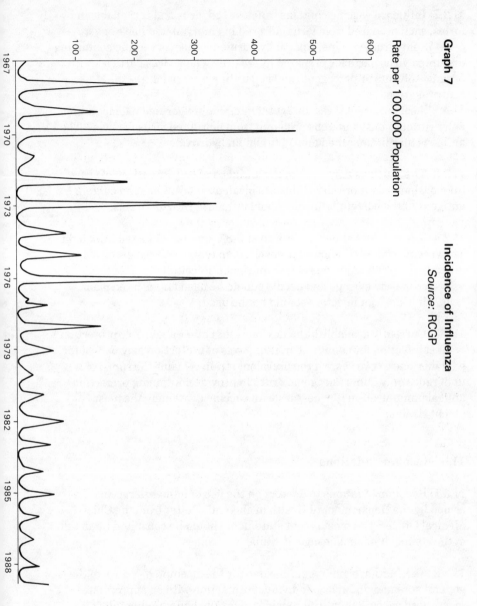

Rate per 100,000 Population

11.2.2 Influenza vaccine contains **inactivated** virus and is available in two forms, each prepared from virus cultured in embryonated hen's eggs.

a. "Split virus" vaccine, a partially purified influenza vaccine containing disrupted virus particles prepared by treating whole virus particles with organic solvents or detergents and separating by zonal ultra-centrifugation.

b. "Surface antigen" vaccine, containing highly purified haemaglutinin and neuraminidase antigens prepared from disrupted virus particles. The antigens may be adsorbed on to aluminium hydroxide.

11.2.3 The vaccines may contain the antigens of only one strain of virus (monovalent) but more commonly are bivalent or trivalent, and contain antigens of the current influenza A and influenza B virus strains.

11.2.4 The vaccines should be stored at 2-8°C and be protected from light. The vaccine should be allowed to reach room temperature before being given by deep subcutaneous or intramuscular injection.

a. A separate syringe and needle should be used for each recipient.

b. Multidose jet injectors should not be used.

11.2.5 Currently available influenza vaccines confer about 70% protection against infection for about a year. Low levels of protection may persist for a further one to two years if the prevalent strain remains the same, or undergoes only minor 'antigenic drift'. To provide continuing protection annual immunisation is necessary with vaccine containing the most recent strains.

11.3 Recommendations

11.3.1 Recommendations to doctors on the use of influenza vaccine are issued by the Department of Health in an annual letter from the Chief Medical Officer. The most recent statement should be consulted for details of the composition and dosage of available vaccines.

11.3.2 Vaccination is not recommended for the attempted control of the general spread of influenza. Individual protection with an appropriate inactivated vaccine should be considered for **persons at special risk** provided that vaccine is not contraindicated (11.5). These groups include persons, especially the elderly, suffering from the following conditions:-

a. chronic pulmonary disease
b. chronic heart disease
c. chronic renal disease
d. diabetes, and other less common endocrine disorders
e. conditions involving immunosuppressive therapy.

11.3.3 The vaccine should be considered for elderly persons and children living in residential homes and long-stay hospitals.

11.3.4 To minimise the risk of febrile reactions after influenza vaccine in children, purified surface antigen vaccine should be used. The recommended lower age limit for vaccination of children is four years of age.

11.3.5 Vaccination of Health Service staff is indicated only for those individuals at increased risk owing to medical disorders such as those above. In the event of a pandemic or other major outbreak, advice would be given about vaccination of staff particularly liable to exposure.

11.4 Adverse reactions

11.4.1 Local reactions, consisting of redness and induration at the injection site lasting one to two days may occur in up to a third of recipients, but these are usually mild. Recent influenza virus vaccines have been associated with few side-effects; two types have been described:

a. Fever, malaise, myalgia beginning six to 12 hours after vaccination and persisting one to two days. This occurs more often in children than adults.

b. Immediate responses of an allergic nature resulting in urticaria or respiratory expressions of hypersensitivity. These are very rare.

11.4.2 Adverse reactions to influenza vaccine should be reported to the Committee on Safety of Medicines using the yellow card system.

11.5 Contraindications

See Sections 2.2 and 2.2.1 of General Topics.

11.5.1
   a. Individuals with hypersensitivity to eggs should **not** be
given influenza vaccine as residual egg protein is present in
minute quantities. The vaccine should not be used in persons
hypersensitive to polymyxin or neomycin as traces of these antibiotics may
be present.
   b. **Pregnancy.** Some evidence from past pandemic experience suggests
that influenza in pregnancy is associated with increased risks of maternal
mortality, and congenital malformations and leukaemia in the children.
Other studies have not supported these observations, thus the significance
of influenza during pregnancy is uncertain. There is no evidence that
influenza vaccine prepared from inactivated virus causes damage to the
fetus, but as with other vaccines it should not be given during pregnancy
unless there is a specific risk.

11.6 Management of outbreaks

11.6.1 As transmission of influenza virus is person-to-person via the
respiratory tract, one method of limiting an outbreak is to interrupt the
chain of infection. Influenza has a higher mortality in the elderly and
chronic sick, and contact for them with infected people should be avoided.
Immunisation of contacts during an outbreak is not effective.
Antiviral chemoprophylaxis, such as amantadine hydrochloride, may give
protection against influenza A infection.

11.7 Supplies

Information on current vaccines is given in the latest CMO letter from the
Department of Health. Vaccines are available from:-

Duphar Tel. 0703 472281.
Servier Tel. 02816 2647/2744.
Merieux UK Ltd Tel. 0628 785291.

Immunisation against Infectious Disease

11.8 Bibliography

Immunisation against influenza: rationale and recommendations.
Eickhoff T C.
J Infect Dis 1971; 123, 446-54

A controlled double blind comparison of reactogenicity, immunogenicity and protective efficacy of whole-virus and split-product influenza vaccine in children.
Gross P A et al.
J Infect Dis 1977; 136, 623-632.

Assessment of inactivated influenza A vaccine after three outbreaks of influenza A at Christ's Hospital.
Hoskins T W, Davies J R, et al.
Lancet 1979; (i), 33-35.

Summary of clinical trials of influenza vaccines.
Parkman P D, Galasso G H et al.
J Infect Dis 1976; 134, 100-107.

Vaccination against influenza A.
Tyrell D A J, Smith J W G.
Br Med Bull 1979; 35 (i), 77-85.

Influenza

12 Hepatitis A

12.1 Hepatitis A is transmitted by the faecal oral route generally after the ingestion of contaminated food or drink. The disease is usually milder than hepatitis B and is very seldom fatal but occasional cases of fulminating hepatitis may occur. A chronic carrier state is unknown and chronic liver damage is extremely unlikely. The incubation period is about 15-40 days. Outbreaks occasionally occur in this country although most cases are sporadic. Persons travelling to developing countries may be at greater risk of contracting hepatitis A.

12.2 Human normal immunoglobulin (HNIG) offers protection against infection with hepatitis A and is normally used under the following circumstances:

(i) To close contacts of all ages in order to control outbreaks of hepatitis A in households and in institutions.

Age	Dose
Under ten years	250mg
Ten years and over	500mg

(ii) For travellers abroad to all countries excluding Northern Europe, North America, Australia and New Zealand.

Period abroad	Age	Dose
Two months or less	Under ten years	125mg
	Ten years and over	250mg
Three to five months	Under ten years	250mg
	Ten years and over	500mg

Where practical, persons requesting HNIG for prophylaxis against hepatitis A should be screened for antibodies to assess the need. This is particularly so where repeated administrations of HNIG are likely.

12.3 Human normal immunoglobulin may interfere with the development of active immunity from live virus vaccines. It is therefore wise to administer live virus vaccines at least three weeks before the administration of immunoglobulin. If immunoglobulin has been administered first, then an interval of three months should be observed before administering a live virus vaccine. This does not apply to yellow fever vaccine since HNIG does not contain antibody to this virus. For travellers, if there is insufficient time, the recommended intervals may have to be ignored, especially where oral polio vaccine is concerned.

12.4 Supplies

HNIG from Central Public Health Laboratory Tel. 081-200 6868;
       Public Health Laboratories, England and Wales
       Blood Products Laboratory Tel. 081-953 6191
       Blood Transfusion Service, Scotland

       The Laboratories, Belfast City Hospital Tel.0232 329241

       Immuno Tel.0732 458101 (Gammabulin)
       Kabivitrum Tel.0895 51144 (Kabiglobulin)

Hepatitis A

13. Hepatitis B

13.1 Introduction

13.1.1 Viral hepatitis B usually has an insidious onset with anorexia, vague abdominal discomfort, nausea and vomiting, sometimes arthralgia and rash, which often progresses to jaundice. Fever may be absent or mild. The severity of the disease ranges from inapparent infections, which can only be detected by liver function tests and/or the presence of serological markers of acute HBV infection (eg. HBsAg, anti BHc IgM), to fulminating fatal cases of acute hepatic necrosis. Among cases admitted to hospital the fatality rate is about 1%. The average incubation period is 40-160 days but occasionally can be as long as six to nine months.

13.1.2 The number of overt cases of acute hepatitis B identified in the UK appears to be low, averaging around 1000 reported cases a year. The prevalence of hepatitis B surface antigenaemia (HBsAg) is not known with certainty but is in the order of about one in 500 of the blood donor adult population; often such individuals do not give a history of clinical hepatitis. A proportion of antigen carriers develop chronic hepatitis. Sometimes there is impairment of liver function tests; biopsy findings range from normal to active hepatitis, with or without cirrhosis. The prognosis of the liver disease in such individuals is at present uncertain, but it is known that some will develop hepatocellular carcinoma.

13.1.3 In recent years there has been a sharp decrease in the annual total of acute hepatitis B reports to the Public Health Laboratory Services since the peak of 1,995 reports in 1984. This is particularly associated with a change in the annual number of reports of cases with a history of drug abuse. Whilst the availability of vaccine might have played a role, a more probable explanation is the similarity of the routes of transmission of HBV and HIV, the educational campaigns to prevent spread of HIV and the increased availability of sterile needles and syringes.

See Graph viii Page 99

13.1.4 Certain occupational and other groups are known to be at increased risk of infection (see paragraph 13.3).

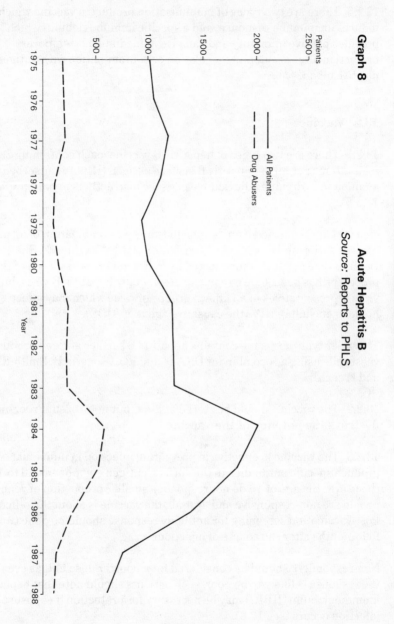

Hepatitis B

Graph 8

Acute Hepatitis B
Source: Reports to PHLS

All Patients
Drug Abusers

Patients

2500

2000

1500

1000

500

1975 1976 1977 1978 1979 1980 1981 1982 1983 1984 1985 1986 1987 1988

Year

Immunisation against Infectious Disease

99

13.1.5 There are two types of immunisation product: a vaccine which induces an immune response, and a specific immunoglobulin which provides passive immunity and can give immediate but temporary protection after accidental inoculation or contamination with antigen positive blood.

13.2 Vaccine

13.2.1 There are two types of hepatitis B vaccine, each containing 20 micrograms per ml of hepatitis B surface antigen (HBsAg) adsorbed on aluminium hydroxide adjuvant (see dosage instructions in paragraph 13.3.8).

One vaccine is purified from human plasma by a combination of ultra-centrifugation and biochemical procedures, (H-B-Vax, Merck, Sharp and Dohme). The product is inactivated by a threefold process; each of these processes has been shown to inactivate not only hepatitis B virus, but also virus representatives of all known groups of virus which may infect humans, including HIV (the causative agent of AIDS).

The other type of vaccine contains hepatitis B surface antigen produced by yeast cells using a recombinant DNA technique, (Engerix B, Smith Kline and French).

13.2.2 The vaccine should be stored at 2-8°C but not frozen. **Freezing destroys the potency of the vaccine.**

13.2.3 The vaccine is effective in preventing infection in individuals who produce specific antibodies to the surface antigen component. 10 to 15% of those over the age of 40 do not respond; a smaller proportion of younger people are non-responsive and, overall, the vaccine is about 90% effective. Post-vaccination screening for antibody response should be done two to four months after the course of injections.

Non-responders should be considered for a booster dose but, as even then the response is likely to be poor, such patients should note that hepatitis B immunoglobulin (HBIG) may be necessary for protection if exposure to infection occurs (see 13.8).

Immunisation against Infectious Disease

Patients who are immunodeficient or on immunosuppressive therapy may respond less well than healthy individuals and may require larger doses of vaccine or an additional dose (see 13.3.8).

The duration of antibody persistence is not known precisely but is of the order of three to five years. Advice on the need for further booster doses cannot yet be formulated, but individuals who are at high risk may wish to determine their antibody level periodically. If this falls below 50Iu/L the need for a booster dose must be considered.Suitable intervals for testing antibody levels are at one year and five years after the primary course and post-vaccination test.

13.3 Recommendations

13.3.1 Vaccination should be considered for the groups of individuals discussed in the succeeding paragraphs under the headings "Health Care Personnel", "Patients and Family Contacts", and "Other Indications for Immunisation". It should be offered to those at highest risk as described in 13.3.5, although this list should not be regarded as exclusive.

13.3.2 Immunisation takes up to six months to confer adequate protection. This should be kept in mind when considering the need for individuals to have the vaccine. It is especially relevant in the case of new students and trainees.

NB. It is important that vaccination against hepatitis B does not encourage relaxation of good infection-control procedures.

13.3.3 The vaccine should **not** be given to individuals known to be hepatitis B surface antigen positive, or to patients with acute hepatitis B, since in the former case it would be unnecessary and, in the latter, ineffective. Intimate contacts of individuals suffering from acute hepatitis B and sexual contacts of highly infectious carriers should be treated by passive immunisation (see 13.8) followed by active immunisation (which can be commenced simultaneously).

13.3.4 Hepatitis B vaccine **may** be given to HIV positive individuals (see 2.4, 13.2.3, 13.8).

Screening for HBV markers prior to vaccination may sometimes be considered in a population where the antibody prevalence is expected to be high and will also depend on the local cost and availability of screening tests.

13.3.5 Health care personnel

Doctors, dentists, nurses, midwives and others, including students and trainees, who have direct contact with patients or their body fluids, or are likely to experience frequent parenteral exposure to blood or blood-contaminated secretions and excretions, should be considered as being at high risk.

Groups particularly to be considered in this high risk category are:

a. Those health care personnel and others who are at risk and directly involved over a period of six months or more in patient care in institutions or units for the mentally handicapped.

b. Those directly involved in patient care over a period of six months or more working in units giving treatment to known carriers of hepatitis B infection.

c. Laboratory workers, mortuary technicians.

d. Health care personnel on secondment to work in areas of the world with a high prevalence of hepatitis B infection, if they are to be directly involved in patient care.

13.3.6 Patients and family contacts

a. Patients on entry into institutions or units dealing with the mentally handicapped, where appropriate.

b. The immune response to the current hepatitis B vaccines is poorer in immunocompromised patients and those over 40. For example, only about 60% of patients undergoing treatment by maintenance haemodialysis develop anti-HBs. It is suggested, therefore, that patients with chronic renal damage be immunised as soon as it appears likely that they will ultimately require treatment by maintenance haemodialysis or renal transplant.

c. The spouses or other sexual partners of carriers of hepatitis B if the potential vaccinee is negative for hepatitis B surface antigen or surface antibody.

Immunisation against Infectious Disease

d. Haemophiliacs and those receiving regular blood transfusions or blood products.

13.3.7 Other indications for immunisation

Consideration should also be given to members of the following groups, and it should be noted here that if the recommended precautions to protect against HIV infection were taken, the risk of spread of HBV would be considerably reduced. High risk groups requiring vaccination after exposure are described under post-exposure protection (13.8).

a. Police and Emergency Services

The statistics of the incidence of hepatitis B do not show that, in general, members of the police, ambulance, rescue services and staff of custodial institutions are at greater risk than the general population. Nevertheless, there may be individuals within these occupations who are at higher risk and who should be considered for vaccination. Such a selection has to be decided locally by the occupational health services, or following other medical advice as appropriate.

b. Persons visiting other countries

For short visits abroad by the ordinary tourist or business person who will not indulge in high risk activities, the need for vaccination is questionable. It should however be considered before visits to regions where hepatitis B is endemic for:-

(i) Those planning to work or live there for lengthy periods where there may be a risk of acquiring infection from medical procedures using inadequately sterilised equipment.
(ii) Those who will be involved in the care of patients in such areas.

c **Morticians and embalmers.**

d **Individuals who frequently change sexual partners, particularly prostitutes and male homosexuals.**

e **Inmates of long-term custodial institutions.**

f **Parenteral drug abusers.**

Immunisation against Infectious Disease   103

13.3.8 Recommended dosage for primary immunisation

The basic immunisation regimen consists of three doses of vaccine, with the first dose at the elected date, the second dose one month later and the third dose at six months after the first dose.

The recombinant vaccine has also been used where more rapid immunisation is required, for example with travellers when the third dose may be given at two months after the initial dose with a booster dose at 12 months.

The vaccine should normally be given intramuscularly. The injection should be given in the deltoid region, though the anterolateral thigh is the preferred site for infants. The buttock must not be used because vaccine efficacy may be reduced.

In patients with haemophilia, the intradermal or subcutaneous route may be used.

Doctors are however advised that until such time as the manufacturers apply for and are granted variations to their product licenses for the intradermal route of administration, the use of this route would be on their own personal responsibility.

13.3.9 Dosage schedule

Reference should be made to the manufacturers latest data sheet for details. The paediatric dosage recommendations for the two available vaccines differ slightly.

Engerix B	children from birth to 12 years	0.5ml (10 micrograms) intramuscularly
	adults	1.0ml (20 micrograms) intramuscularly
H-B Vax	newborn infants and children under ten years	0.5ml (10 micrograms) intramuscularly
	adults and children over ten years	1.0ml (20 micrograms) intramuscularly
	immunocompromised and dialysis patients	2.0ml (40 micrograms) given as two 1.0ml doses at different sites.

The intradermal dose (but see 13.3.8) is 0.1ml (two micrograms).

13.4 Adverse reactions

13.4.1 Hepatitis B vaccines are generally well tolerated and the most common adverse reactions are soreness and redness at the injection site. Injection intradermally may produce a persisting nodule at the site of the injection, sometimes with local pigmentation changes. Other less common reactions which have been reported include fever, rash, malaise and an influenza-like syndrome, arthralgia and myalgia.

13.4.2 It is important that adverse reactions should be reported to the Committee on Safety of Medicines by the yellow card system.

13.5 Pregnancy

Hepatitis B infection in pregnant women may result in severe disease for the mother and chronic infection of the newborn. Vaccination should not be withheld from a pregnant woman if she is in a high risk category.

13.6 Effect of vaccination on carriers

The vaccine produces neither therapeutic nor adverse effects on carriers of hepatitis B.

13.7 Contraindications

Vaccination should be postponed in individuals suffering from febrile infections.

13.8 Post-exposure protection

13.8.1 Specific hepatitis B immunoglobulin (HBIG) is available for passive protection and is normally used in combination with hepatitis B vaccine to confer passive/active immunity after exposure.

13.8.2 Whenever immediate protection is required, immunisation with the vaccine should be combined with simultaneous administration of hepatitis B immunoglobulin (HBIG) at a different site. It has been shown that passive immunisation with HBIG does not suppress an active immune response. A single dose of HBIG (usually 500 Iu for adults; 200 Iu for the newborn) is sufficient for healthy individuals. If infection has already occurred at the time of the first immunisation, virus multiplication is unlikely to be inhibited completely, but severe illness and, most importantly, the development of the carrier state of HBV may be prevented in many individuals, particularly in infants born to carrier mothers.

13.8.3 Groups requiring post-exposure protection are:-

a. Infants born to mothers who are persistent carriers of hepatitis B surface antigen, particularly if hepatitis e antigen (HBeAg) is detectable or its antibody (anti-HBe) is not, or hepatitis B virus DNA is detectable. The nature and size of the risk at birth varies from persistent carriage in 80-90% of infants of HBeAg positive mothers to the less frequent occurrence of hepatitis B infection in infants of anti-HBe positive mothers, frequently in relation to the ethnic group of the mother.

Immunisation against Infectious Disease

It is most important to identify the infants at risk, and antenatal patients in high risk categories should be screened. These include:

(i) All ethnic groups other than Caucasian, though Caucasians from Southern and Eastern Europe should also be considered.
(ii) All those with a personal or family history of occupation suggestive of increased risk of exposure to hepatitis B virus (HBV).

b. Infants born to mothers HBsAg positive as a result of recent infection, particularly if HBeAg is detectable or anti-HBe is not.

Active/passive immunisation with vaccine and hepatitis B immunoglobulin is recommended for infants at risk. The first dose of vaccine should be given at birth or as soon as possible thereafter, and preferably within 12 hours and not later than 48 hours. Hepatitis B immunoglobulin should be given at a contralateral site at the same time; arrangements should be made well in advance.

c. Persons who are accidentally inoculated, or who contaminate the eye or mouth or fresh cuts or abrasions of skin, with blood from a known HBsAg positive person. Individuals who sustain such accidents should wash the affected area well and seek medical advice. Advice about prophylaxis after such accidents should be obtained by telephone from the nearest Public Health Laboratory. Advice following accidental exposure may also be obtained from the Hospital Control of Infection Officer or the Occupational Health Services.

Health care workers who have already been successfully vaccinated should be given a booster dose of vaccine unless they are known to have adequate protective levels of antibodies.

d. Sexual consorts, (and in some circumstances a family contact judged to be at high risk) of individuals suffering from acute hepatitis B, and who are seen within one week of onset of jaundice in the contact.

13.8.4 There is no evidence associating the administration of intramuscular immunoglobulin, either normal or specific, with acquisition of HIV infection. Not only does the processing of the plasma from which these immunoglobulins are prepared render them safe, but the screening of blood donations is now routine practice.

Hepatitis B

13.8.5 Dosage: Hepatitis B immunoglobulin is available in 2ml ampoules containing 200 Iu and 5ml ampoules containing 500 Iu.

Newborn 200 Iu as soon as possible and not later than 48 hours after birth.

Children:

0-4 years	200Iu)	preferably within 48 hours
5-9 years	300Iu)	and not later than a week
10 years or more	500Iu)	after exposure
Adult	500Iu)	

13.9 Supplies of Hepatitis B immunoglobulin.

Public Health Laboratory Service, either from the Communicable Disease Surveillance Centre (Tel: 081-200 6868) or via local Public Health Laboratories. Hepatitis B immunoglobulin is held in Scotland by the Blood Transfusion Service:

Aberdeen	(0224) 681818
Dundee	(0382) 645166
Edinburgh	(031) 2297291
Glasgow	(0698) 373315/8
Inverness	(0463) 234151

Hepatitis B immunoglobulin is held in Northern Ireland by the Regional Virus Laboratory, Royal Victoria Hospital, Belfast.
Tel: (0232) 240503.

Note: Supplies of this product are limited and demands should be restricted to patients in whom there is a clear indication for its use.

13.10 Supplies of Hepatitis B Vaccine.

The following Hepatitis B vaccines are available:

H-B-Vax	Merck Sharp and Dohme Ltd. Tel. 0992 467272
Engerix B	Smith Kline and French. Tel. 0707 325111.

Immunisation against Infectious Disease

14 Rabies

14.1 Introduction

14.1.1 Rabies is an acute viral infection resulting in encephalomyelitis. The onset is insidious. Early symptoms may include paraesthesiae around the site of the wound, fever, headache and malaise. The disease may present in one of two ways; hydrophobia, hallucinations, and maniacal behaviour progressing to paralysis and coma, or an ascending flaccid paralysis and sensory disturbance. Rabies is almost always fatal, with death resulting from respiratory paralysis. The incubation period is generally two to eight weeks, but may range from nine days to two years.

14.1.2 Infection is usually via the bite of a rabid animal, but transmission of the virus can also occur through mucous membranes, though not through intact skin. Person-to-person spread of the disease is extremely rare, but instances of transmission by corneal graft have been reported. No indigenous human rabies has been reported in the United Kingdom since 1902 although cases occur in persons infected abroad. The disease occurs in all continents except Australasia and Antarctica. Rabies in animals has spread throughout a great part of Central and Western Europe since 1945 and continues to advance westwards. In Europe foxes are predominantly infected but many other animals become infected including dogs and cats, cattle, horses, badgers, martens and deer. The prevention of rabies spreading to the UK depends on the control of imported animals. Individuals at high risk of exposure, such as animal handlers, should be given pre-exposure vaccine (see 14.3.1). Rabies vaccine is used for pre-exposure protection, whilst both vaccine and rabies specific immunoglobulin may be needed for rabies post-exposure treatment.

14.2 Vaccine

14.2.1 The vaccine currently available is a human diploid cell vaccine (HDCV). It is a freeze dried suspension of Wistar rabies virus strain PM/WI 38 1503-3M cultured on human diploid cells and inactivated by beta-propiolactone. For post-exposure treatment the potency of the reconstituted vaccine should be not less than 2.5 × the International

Immunisation against Infectious Disease   109

Standard per 1ml dose. The freeze-dried vaccine should be stored at 4°C and used immediately after re-constitution with the diluent supplied. It may be given by deep subcutaneous, intramuscular or intradermal injection; post-vaccination antibody may not be apparent until the tenth day of a course. The antibody response may be poor if the gluteal region is used for injection.

14.2.2 Rabies-specific immunoglobulin

Passive immunisation with human rabies immunoglobulin (HRIG) provides rapid immune protection for a short period and can be used in combination with HDCV in post-exposure treatment to cover the delay associated with active immunisation. HRIG is obtained from the plasma of vaccinated human donors.

14.3 Recommendations

14.3.1 HDCV may be used for pre-exposure prophylaxis and post-exposure treatment (see under Management of Cases). Pre-exposure vaccination should be offered to those employed in the following categories:-

   a. At animal quarantine premises for imported animals and zoological establishments.
   b. As carrying agents authorised to carry imported animals.
   c. At approved research and acclimatisation centres where primates and other imported animals are housed.
   d. At national ports of entry where contact with imported animals is likely (e.g. Customs and Excise Officers).
   e. As veterinary and technical staff of the Ministry of Agriculture, Fisheries and Food (MAFF) and Department of Agriculture and Fisheries for Scotland (DAFS).
   f. As inspectors appointed by local authorities under the Diseases of Animals Act, or employed otherwise who, by reason of their employment, encounter increased risk.
   g. In laboratories handling rabies virus.
   h. As health workers who come into close contact with a patient with rabies.
   i. As workers in enzootic areas where they may be at special risk (eg veterinary staff or zoologists).

All such persons at occupational risk at home and abroad are entitled to rabies vaccine free from the NHS.

Rabies vaccine may be requested as a prophylactic measure by travellers and those living or working abroad but is not available free from the NHS under these circumstances. Travellers who wish to do so can obtain vaccine on payment.

14.3.2 For pre-exposure protection, two doses of vaccine each of 1.0ml should be given four weeks apart by deep subcutaneous or intramuscular injection in the deltoid region. A reinforcing dose is given after 12 months. Additional reinforcing doses are given every one to three years depending on the risk of exposure, and also following exposure to possible rabies. When more than one person is to be vaccinated the vaccine may be administered in smaller doses (0.1ml) by the intradermal route with the same time intervals as above. It is emphasised that intradermal vaccination is reliable **only if the whole of the 0.1ml dose is properly given into the dermis**. Those not experienced in intradermal technique should give a full dose by intramuscular injection. Staff who are engaged in the care of a patient with rabies may be rapidly immunised by receiving 0.1ml of vaccine intradermally in each limb (0.4ml in all) on the first day of exposure to the patient. The use of the intradermal route is at the doctor's own responsibility as this is not covered by the manufacturer's Product Licence.

14.3.3 Many authorities recommend that a serological test should be carried out on all people receiving rabies vaccine for pre-exposure immunisation, to ensure that they have responded to the initial course of rabies vaccine.

14.3.4 Should an outbreak of rabies in animals occur in the United Kingdom and a rabies-infected area be declared, vaccination would need to be offered, as appropriate, to those persons directly involved in control measures, and to veterinary surgeons and their ancillary staff working within the infected area.

14.4 Adverse reactions

14.4.1 HDCV may cause local reactions such as redness, swelling or pain at the site of injection within 24-48 hours of administration. Systemic reactions such as headache, fever, muscle aches, vomiting, and urticarial rashes have been reported. Anaphylactic shock has been reported from the USA and Guillain-Barré syndrome from Norway.

14.4.2 Suspected adverse reactions should be reported to the Committee on Safety of Medicines using the yellow card system.

14.5 Contraindications

14.5.1 There are no specific contraindications to HDCV, although if there were evidence of hypersensitivity, subsequent doses should not be given, except in the case of treatment.

14.5.2 Pre-exposure vaccine should only be given to pregnant women if the risk of exposure to rabies is high.

14.6 Management of persons exposed to possible rabies

14.6.1 For travellers returning to this country (see 14.1.2) who report an exposure to an animal abroad, treatment should be started while enquiries are made about the prevalence of rabies in the country concerned, and where possible, the condition of the biting animal. Information should be sought from PHLS Virus Reference Laboratory, London (081-200 4400); in Scotland, the Communicable Diseases (Scotland) Unit (041-946 7120); in Northern Ireland, DHSS (0232 650111).

14.6.2 Treatment should be started as soon as possible:

    a. Thorough cleansing of the wound by scrubbing with soap and water under a running tap for five minutes.

    b. Active and, if indicated, passive immunisation.

14.6.3 HRIG should be given immediately (day 0). The recommended dose is 20 IU/Kg body weight, half of which should be thoroughly infiltrated into the area of the wound and the rest given intramuscularly. Local pain and low grade fever may follow the administration of HRIG, but no serious adverse reactions have been reported.

14.6.4 1.0ml of HDCV should be given by deep subcutaneous or

Immunisation against Infectious Disease

intramuscular injection on days 0, 3, 7, 14, 30 and 90. (Day 0 is the day the patient receives the first dose). The vaccine should be given into the deltoid region, or in a child, the anterolateral aspect of the thigh.

14.6.5 WHO recommendations for treatment are given in the WHO Expert Committee Report (see 14.10).

14.6.6 For a previously vaccinated person, a modified course of post-exposure vaccine may be given following a bite by a possibly rabid animal. **Advice should be obtained from the Virus Reference Laboratory, Central Public Health Laboratory, Colindale, London(081-200 4400).**

14.6.7 Human rabies is a notifiable disease. In the event of a case of human rabies, the Medical Officer for Environmental Health (in Scotland the Chief Administrative Medical Officer) should be informed. Detailed advice on management appears in the "Memorandum on Rabies" issued by the DHSS and SHHD in 1977.

14.7 Supplies

14.7.1

a. Human diploid cell vaccine (HDCV) is manufactured by Institut Merieux, France, and is available from Merieux UK Tel. 0628 785291.

HDCV for persons in categories 14.3.1 is supplied by DOH and is available from the PHLS Virus Reference Laboratory, Tel. 081-200 4400. For persons not in these categories for whom it is not available on NHS prescription it should be obtained from commercial sources: Merieux UK Limited, Maidenhead, Berks. (Tel. 0628 785291).

b. For post-exposure use, emergency supplies are also held in several other centres. Information may be obtained from Virus Reference Laboratory, (Tel. 081 200 4400).

c. Human rabies immunoglobulin (HRIG) is manufactured by Blood Products Laboratory and supplied through some Public Health Laboratories (see b. above).

d. Supply Centres in Scotland for HDCV and HRIG are listed in the SHHD Memorandum on Rabies.

Immunisation against Infectious Disease   113

14.8 Immunoglobulin — rabies specific immunoglobulin (HRIG)

HRIG is used after exposure to rabies to provide rapid protection until rabies vaccine, which should be given at the same time, becomes effective.

Dose. 20 IU/Kg body weight. Up to half the dose is infiltrated in and around the wound after thorough cleansing and the rest is given by intramuscular injection.

14.9 Supplies

HRIG is available in 1ml ampoules containing 500 IU.

Central Public Health Laboratory, Tel. 081 200 6868
(Virus Reference Laboratory)

The Laboratories, Belfast City Hospital Tel. 0232 329241

14.10 Bibliography

WHO Expert Committee on Rabies, 7th report.
Technical Report Series, 709 WHO, Geneva 1984.

Immunisation against Infectious Disease

15 Cholera

15.1 Introduction

15.1.1 Cholera is an acute intestinal disease caused by an enterotoxin produced by *Vibrio cholerae*, Serogroup 01, of the classical and El Tor biotypes. Cholera is characterised by sudden onset of profuse watery stools, occasional vomiting, rapid dehydration, metabolic acidosis and circulatory collapse. Over 50% of the most severe cases if untreated may die within a few hours of onset; if treated correctly, mortality is less than 1%. Mild cases with only moderate diarrhoea may occur. Asymptomatic infections are many times more frequent than those with symptoms especially with El Tor cholera. The incubation period is between two and five days but may be only a few hours.

15.1.2 The last indigenous case of cholera was reported in 1893. Between 1970 and 1987, 51 imported cases of cholera with two deaths were reported in England and Wales. Further importation is likely, but the risk of an outbreak is very small in any country with modern sanitation and water supplies, and high standards of food hygiene.

15.1.3 Infection is acquired from contaminated water, shellfish or other food. Even in endemic areas the risk to tourists is very small.

15.1.4 Cholera vaccine is of limited use. In endemic areas, the vaccine has been shown to reduce the incidence of overt disease by only 50%; it also fails to prevent people becoming asymptomatic carriers. Whilst the World Health Organisation (WHO) no longer recommends cholera vaccination for travel to or from cholera infected areas, some countries still require evidence of vaccination six days to six months before entry. It is for this reason, and the fact that vaccination may confer some personal protection, that cholera vaccine is available. Travellers should consult the relevant embassy for up-to-date information.

15.2 Vaccine

15.2.1 Cholera vaccine consists of a heat-killed, phenol-preserved mixed suspension of the Inaba and Ogawa serotypes of Vibrio cholerae, serovar 01. The vaccine is effective against both the classical and the El Tor biotypes. The protection conferred persists for three to six months, but is minimal a year after the last dose.

15.2.2 The vaccine should be stored at 2-8°C. It has a tendency, on standing, to settle out in a gelatinous form. Vigorous shaking will yield a homogeneous suspension suitable for injection. Any partly used multi-dose containers should be discarded at the end of the vaccination session.

15.3 Recommendations

15.3.1 Cholera vaccine is indicated for the following:

a. People travelling to countries which require evidence of cholera vaccination. Travellers should enquire from the relevant Embassy or High Commissioner's office for current requirements. An international certificate of vaccination is no longer required by international regulations but some countries require a medical certificate. This is valid for six months beginning six days after the first dose, or the date of re-vaccination.
b. People travelling to countries or areas where cholera is endemic or epidemic, especially if they will be living in unhygienic conditions.

15.3.2 Cholera vaccine is **not** indicated in the control of the spread of infection or in the management of contacts of imported cases.

15.3.3. Because of the low vaccine efficacy, vaccinees should be told that the best protection against cholera, as well as against other enteric diseases is to avoid food and water which might be contaminated.

15.3.4 A single dose of vaccine may be sufficient to satisfy the regulations of those countries still requiring proof of cholera vaccination for entry. Cholera vaccine is not recommended for children under one year of age.

15.3.5 Cholera vaccine **may** be given to HIV positive individuals.

15.3.6 Primary immunisation consists of two doses of vaccine given by deep subcutaneous or intramuscular injection, separated by a period of at least one week and preferably one month. A booster dose is recommended every six months to maintain immunity. When more than six months have

Immunisation against Infectious Disease

elapsed since the last dose, a single dose is sufficient to boost immunity.

15.3.7 The recommended doses for primary and booster immunisations are:

Deep subcutaneous or intramuscular injection

Age	First dose	All subsequent doses
1-5 years	0.1ml	0.3ml
5-10 years	0.3ml	0.5ml
Over 10 years	0.5ml	1.0ml

The intradermal route is not recommended as there is insufficient evidence of protective efficacy.

15.4 Adverse reactions

15.4.1 Cholera vaccination will occasionally cause some local tenderness and redness at the injection site lasting one to two days. This may be accompanied by fever, malaise and headache. Serious reactions are rare.

15.4.2 Serious reactions should be reported to the Committee on Safety of Medicines using the yellow card system.

15.5 Contraindications

15.5.1
   a. The vaccine should not be given to anyone suffering from febrile illness.

   b. Although there is no information to suggest that cholera vaccine is unsafe during pregnancy, it should only be given when this is unavoidable, ie required for travel.

   c. Repeated vaccinations may result in the development of hypersensitivity.

   d. A severe reaction to cholera vaccination is a contraindication to further doses.

15.6 Management of outbreaks

15.6.1 Cholera vaccine has **no role** in the management of contacts of any cases, or in controlling the spread of infection. Sources of infection should be identified and appropriate measures taken. Contacts should maintain high standards of personal hygiene to avoid becoming infected. Control of the disease is based on public health measures rather than vaccination.

15.7 Supplies

15.7.1 Vials of 1.5ml and 10ml are available from the Wellcome Foundation Ltd Tel: Crewe (0270) 583151.

15.8 Bibliography

Comparative study of reactions and serological response to cholera vaccines in a controlled field trial conducted in the USSR.
Burgasov P N et al.
Bull. WHO 1976; 54 (2): 163-170.

A controlled field trial of the effectiveness of intradermal and subcutaneous administration of cholera vaccine.
Philippines Cholera Committee.
Bull. WHO 1973; 49, 389-394.

Efficacy of vaccination of family contacts of cholera cases.
Sommer A, Khan M, Mosley W H.
Lancet 1973; (i), 1230-1232.

16 Typhoid

16.1 Introduction

16.1.1 Typhoid and paratyphoid fevers are systemic infections caused by bacteria of the Salmonella genus. This genus comprises almost 2000 serotypes, most of which rarely give rise to systemic invasion and usually cause only gastro-enteritis or 'food poisoning'. However, *S.typhi, S.paratyphi* A, B and C and occasionally other salmonella species may produce systemic infection with prolonged pyrexia, prostration and the characteristic clinical picture of 'enteric' fever. The incubation period, which depends on the size of the infecting dose, is usually one to three weeks. Whilst all cases of typhoid and paratyphoid discharge bacilli during their illness, about 10% of typhoid cases continue to excrete for three months and 2-5% become permanent carriers; the likelihood of becoming a chronic carrier increases with age, especially in females.

16.1.2 Salmonella typhi is transmitted mainly by food and drink that has been contaminated with excreta of a human case or carrier. Examples of sources of outbreaks include canned corned beef (Aberdeen 1964), water supplies (Zermatt 1963) and shellfish contaminated by infected water or sewage. Typhoid is now predominantly a disease of countries where water or food supplies are liable to faecal contamination. In 1938 there were nearly 1000 notifications and 144 deaths in England and Wales attributable to typhoid but since 1960 the annual incidence has remained between about 100 and 200 notified cases. Over 80% of the cases acquire infection abroad, principally in the Indian sub-continent.

16.1.3 Combined typhoid and paratyphoid A and B vaccine is no longer available; there is thus no vaccine against paratyphoid fever.

16.2 Vaccine

16.2.1 The monovalent vaccine contains heat-killed, phenol-preserved *S.typhi* organisms at a concentration of not less than 1000 million/ml. One injection gives around 70-80% protection which fades after one year. Doses at an interval of four to six weeks give protection for three years or more.

Immunisation against Infectious Disease 119

Vaccine efficacy is related to the size of the infecting dose encountered after vaccination.

16.2.2 The vaccine should be stored at 2-8°C. Any partly used multi-dose containers should be discarded at the end of the vaccination session.

16.2.3 Typhoid vaccine may be given by deep subcutaneous or intramuscular injection. The intradermal route is not recommended as there is insufficient evidence of protective efficacy.

16.3 Recommendations

16.3.1 Routine typhoid vaccination is not recommended.

It is advised for:

Laboratory workers handling specimens which may contain typhoid organisms.

It should be considered for:

All persons travelling abroad, with the exception of those going to Canada, USA, Australia, New Zealand and Europe.

It is not recommended for contacts of a known typhoid carrier.

16.3.2 The basic course of vaccination consists of two doses separated by four to six weeks. (The Ministry of Defence advise a third dose after six months)

a. **Adults and children over ten years**

Deep subcutaneous/intramuscular

Basic 1	0.5ml
2	0.5ml
Reinforcement	0.5ml (every 3 years)

Immunisation against Infectious Disease

b. Children — one to ten years

Deep subcutaneous/intramuscular

Basic 1	0.25ml
2	0.25ml
Reinforcement	0.25ml (every 3 years)

16.3.3 Although two doses of vaccine are recommended, one dose is effective for a short period. Typhoid vaccine is not recommended for infants under one year as the risk of infection in infants is low. Under conditions of continued or repeated exposure to infection, a reinforcing dose of vaccine should be given every three years.

16.3.4 Typhoid vaccine **may** be given to HIV positive individuals in the absence of contraindications.

16.4 Adverse reactions

16.4.1 Typhoid vaccine commonly produces local reactions such as redness, swelling, pain and tenderness which may appear after two or three hours and persist for a few days. Systemic reactions include malaise, nausea, headache or pyrexia, which usually disappear within 36 hours. Neurological complications have been described but are rare. Reactions are especially common after repeated injections of typhoid vaccine, and are often more marked in persons over 35 years.

16.4.2 Severe reactions should be reported to the Committee on Safety of Medicines using the yellow card system.

16.5 Contraindications

16.5.1 a. Vaccination of children under one year of age is not advised because of the risk of adverse reactions, the relatively low incidence of typhoid in this age group and the relatively mild course of the disease in infants.
b. Typhoid vaccine should not be given to subjects with acute febrile illness.

Immunisation against Infectious Disease 121

c. Typhoid vaccine is not recommended during an outbreak of typhoid fever in the UK as no immediate protection is afforded by the vaccine. There is also some possibility of temporarily increasing susceptibility to infection. Moreover the vaccine renders the diagnosis of suspected illness more difficult because of interference with serological tests.

d. Repeated injections of typhoid vaccine increase the risk of hypersensitivity. Re-vaccination of fully immunised adults should only be required for those travelling to or staying in endemic areas under conditions of poor hygiene.

e. Although there is no information to suggest that typhoid vaccine is unsafe during pregnancy, it should only be used if clear indication exists.

16.6 Management of outbreaks

16.6.1 It is important that the Medical Officer for Environmental Health (MOEH) or, in Scotland, the Chief Administrative Medical Officer (CAMO) should be informed immediately whenever a patient is suspected of suffering from typhoid without waiting for laboratory confirmation.

16.6.2 Early identification of the source of infection is vital in containing this disease. Household contacts of cases, (that is, those exposed to faeces or vomit of a case, or to the same source), should be excluded from work **if they are involved in food handling,** until at least two, and in some cases three, negative faecal cultures have been obtained. The need for strict personal hygiene should be stressed.

16.7 Supplies

16.7.1 Vials of 1.5ml are available from the Wellcome Foundation Limited. Tel: Crewe (0270) 583151.

16.8 Bibliography

A seven year field trial of two typhoid vaccines in Guyana.
Ashcroft M T et al.
Lancet 1967: (ii), 1056-1059.

Immunisation against Infectious Disease

The present status of field and laboratory studies of typhoid and
paratyphoid vaccines.
Cvjetanovic B, Uemara K.
Bull. WHO 1965: 32, 29-36.

The changing pattern of foodborne disease in England and Wales.
Galbraith N S, Barrett N J, Sockett P N.
Pub. Hlth 1987. 101; 319-328.

Duration of post vaccination anti-typhoid immunity according to the results
of strictly controlled field trials.
Hejfec L B.
J. Hyg. Epid. Microbiol. Imm. 1969: 13, 154-165.

Intradermal versus subcutaneous immunisation with typhoid vaccine.
Iwarson S, Larrson P.
J. Hyg. Camb. (1980): 84, 11-16.

Typhoid

17 Anthrax

17.1 Anthrax is an acute bacterial disease affecting the skin and, rarely, the lungs or gastro-intestinal tract. It is caused by a spore bearing aerobic bacillus, *Bacillus anthraces* and is primarily a disease of herbivorous animals. In the UK it is rare - nine cases notified in the last ten years - and only affects workers exposed to infected hides, wool, hair, bristle, bone, bonemeal, feeding stuffs and carcasses. Spores may survive for many years, and new areas of infection may develop through the use of infected animal feed. Prevention depends on controlling anthrax in livestock and by disinfecting imported animal products. Processing of hides, wool and bone by tanning, dyeing, carbonising or acid treatment ensures that the final product carries no risk of infection. Bonemeal used as horticultural fertiliser may rarely contain anthrax spores; those handling it in bulk should wear impervious gloves which should be destroyed after use.

17.2 Vaccine

Human anthrax vaccine is the alum precipitate of the antigen found in the sterile filtrate of the Sterne strain cultures of *Bacillus anthraces*, with thiomersal preservative. It must be kept at 2-8°C and should be well shaken before being given by intramuscular injection.

17.3 Recommendations

17.3.1 Vaccination against anthrax is recommended **only for workers at risk of exposure to the disease (17.1).** Four injections of 0.5ml should be given, with intervals of three weeks between the first three injections and six months between the third and fourth. Annual reinforcing doses of 0.5ml are advised.

17.3.2 Workers at special risk should wear protective clothing. Adequate washing facilities, ventilation and dust control in hazardous industries should be provided. Prompt reporting and scrupulous medical care of skin abrasions are essential.

17.4 Adverse reactions

17.4.1 These are rare. Mild erythema and swelling lasting up to two days may occur at the site of the injection. Occasionally regional lymphadenopathy, mild fever and urticaria may develop.

17.4.2 Severe reactions should be reported to the Committee on Safety of Medicines using the yellow card system.

17.5 Contraindications

There are no specific contraindications. A local or general reaction to the first injection does not necessarily indicate a predisposition to reactions following subsequent injections.

17.6 Management of outbreaks

17.6.1 All cases of anthrax should be notified; an attempt should be made to confirm the diagnosis bacteriologically and the source of infection should be investigated. Penicillin is the treatment of choice. Skin lesions should be covered; any discharge or soiled articles should be disinfected. Anthrax vaccine has no role in the management of a case or outbreak.

17.7 Supplies

Anthrax vaccine is available from:
Public Health Laboratory Service:
Communicable Disease Surveillance Centre. Tel 081 200 6868
Centre for Applied Microbiology and Research. Tel 0980 610391
Cardiff Tel. 0222 755944
Leeds Tel. 0532 645011
Liverpool Tel. 051 525 2323

Scotland: Bridge of Earn Tel. 073 881 2331
Law Tel. 0698 351100
Borders General Hospital. Tel. 0896 4333

Anthrax

Northern Ireland:
The Laboratories, Belfast City Hospital Tel 0232 329 241

17.8 Bibliography

Vaccine against anthrax.
Editorial.
BMJ 1965: ii; 717-8.

The epidemiology of anthrax.
James D G.
J Antimicrob. Chemother. 1976; 2(4); 319-20.

Thoroughly modern anthrax.
Turnbull P C.
Abstracts of Hygiene, Bureau Hyg & Trop. Dis. 1986; 61(9).

Anthrax

18 Smallpox and Vaccinia

18.1 In December 1979 the Global Commission for the Certification of Smallpox Eradication declared the world free of smallpox and this declaration was ratified by the World Health Assembly in May 1980.

THERE IS THUS NO INDICATION FOR SMALLPOX VACCINATION FOR ANY INDIVIDUAL WITH THE EXCEPTION OF SOME LABORATORY STAFF AND SPECIFIC WORKERS AT IDENTIFIABLE RISK (18.2).

18.2 Recommendations

Workers in laboratories where pox viruses (such as vaccinia) are handled, and others whose work involves an identifiable risk of exposure to pox virus, should be advised of the possible risk and vaccination should be considered. Detailed guidance for laboratory staff has been prepared by the Advisory Committee on Dangerous Pathogens and the Advisory Committee on Genetic Manipulation (in Press). Further advice on the need for vaccination and contraindications should be obtained from Public Health Laboratory Service Virus Reference Laboratory Tel 081 200 4400; if vaccination is considered desirable, vaccine can be obtained through PHLS on this number.

Smallpox and Vaccinaia

19 Yellow Fever

19.1 Introduction

19.1.1 Yellow fever is an acute viral infection occurring in tropical Africa and S. America; it has never been seen in Asia. It ranges in severity from non-specific symptoms to an illness of sudden onset with fever, vomiting and prostration which may progress to haemorrhage and jaundice. In indigenous populations in endemic areas fatality is about 5%; in non-indigenous individuals and during epidemics fatality may reach 50%. Two epidemiological forms, urban and jungle, are recognised although they are clinically and aetiologically identical. Only a few outbreaks of urban yellow fever have occurred in recent years. The incubation period is two to five days.

19.1.2 Urban yellow fever is spread from infected to susceptible persons by *Aedes aegypti*, a mosquito which lives and breeds in close association with man. Jungle yellow fever is a zoonosis transmitted among non-human hosts (mainly monkeys) by forest mosquitoes which may also bite and infect humans. These may, if subsequently bitten by *Aedes aegypti* become the source of outbreaks of the urban form of the disease.

19.1.3 Preventative measures against urban yellow fever include eradication of Aedes mosquitoes, protection from mosquitoes, and vaccination. Jungle fever can only be prevented by vaccination.

19.2 Vaccine

19.2.1 Yellow fever vaccine is a live attenuated freeze-dried preparation of the 17D strain of yellow fever virus. Each 0.5ml dose contains not less than 1000 mouse LD50 units. It is propagated in leucosis-free chick embryos and contains no more than 2 Iu of neomycin and 5 Iu of polymyxin per dose.

19.2.2 It should be stored at 2-8°C and protected from light. The diluent supplied for use with the vaccine should be stored below 15°C but not frozen. The vaccine should be given by subcutaneous injection within one hour of reconstitution. It is given only at designated centres as listed in 19.9.

Immunisation against Infectious Disease

19.2.3 A single dose correctly given confers immunity in nearly 100% of recipients; immunity persists for at least ten years and may be for life.

19.3 Recommendations

19.3.1 The following should be vaccinated:

a. Laboratory workers handling infected material.

b. Persons aged nine months and over travelling through or living in infected areas. Vaccination under nine months is not recommended but may be performed if exposure to the risk of infection cannot be avoided.

Note. A valid International Certificate of Vaccination is compulsory for entry or travel through endemic areas. Requirements should be checked at the relevant Embassy.

19.3.2 The dose is 0.5ml irrespective of age. The International Certificate is valid for ten years from the tenth day after primary vaccination and immediately after revaccination. For travellers, yellow fever vaccine is only given at centres approved by WHO (see 19.9).

19.3.3 Revaccination every ten years is recommended for travellers to infected areas and laboratory workers at special risk.

19.3.4 Normal human immunoglobulin obtained in the UK is unlikely to contain antibody to the yellow fever virus; the vaccine can therefore be given at the same time as an injection of immunoglobulin for travellers abroad.

19.4 Adverse reactions

19.4.1 Severe reactions are extremely rare. 5-10% of recipients have mild headache, myalgia, low-grade fever or soreness at the injection site five to ten days after vaccination.

19.4.2 The only serious reaction following 17D tissue culture vaccine has been the rare occurrence of encephalitis in young infants.

19.4.3 Severe reactions should be reported to the Committee on Safety of Medicines using the yellow card system.

19.5 Contraindications

19.5.1 The usual contraindications to a live virus vaccine should be observed (see 2.2):

   a. Persons suffering from febrile illness.

   b. Patients receiving high-dose corticosteroid or immunosuppressive treatment, including radiation.

   c. Patients suffering from malignant conditions such as lymphoma, leukaemia, Hodgkin's disease or other tumours of the reticulo-endothelial system, or where the immunological mechanism may be impaired as in hypogammaglobulinaemia.

   d. Pregnant women, because of the theoretical risk of fetal infection. However if a pregnant woman must travel to a high risk area, she should be vaccinated since the risk from yellow fever outweighs that of vaccination.

   e. Persons known to be hypersensitive to neomycin or polymyxin or to have had an anaphylactic reaction to egg. A letter stating that vaccination is contraindicated on these grounds may be acceptable in some countries. Advice should be sought from the appropriate Embassy.

   f. Yellow fever vaccine should not be given to either symptomatic or asymptomatic HIV positive individuals since there is as yet insufficient evidence as to the safety of its use. Travellers should be told of this uncertainty and advised not to be vaccinated unless there are compelling reasons (see Section 2.4.4).

19.5.2 If more than one live vaccine is required, they should either be given at the same time in different sites or with an interval of three weeks between them.

19.5.3 Infants under nine months should only be vaccinated if the risk of yellow fever is unavoidable as there is a very small risk of encephalitis (19.4.2).

Immunisation against Infectious Disease

19.6 There is no risk of transmission from imported cases since the mosquito vector does not occur in the UK.

19.7 Supplies

Manufactured and supplied to designated centres by Wellcome, Tel. 0270 583151.

19.8 Bibliography

The duration of immunity following vaccination with the 17D strain of yellow fever virus.
Fox J P, Cabral A S.
Am. J. Hyg. 1943; 37; 93-120.

Stabilised 17D yellow fever vaccine: dose response studies, clinical reactions and effects on hepatic function.
Freestone D S et al.
J. Biol Stand. 1977: 5(3), 181-6.

Neutralising and HAI antibody to yellow fever 17 years after vaccination with 17D vaccine.
Groot H, Ribeivo R B.
Bull WHO 1962; 27; 699-707.

Yellow Fever

19.9 YELLOW FEVER VACCINATION CENTRES: ENGLAND, WALES, SCOTLAND, NORTHERN IRELAND AND ISLE OF MAN.

Yellow fever vaccination centres managed by health authorities are marked thus (*)

England

Altrincham

Dr M R Underwood
Group Surgery
Normans Place, Off Regent Road
Altrincham
Cheshire WA14 2AV

061 928 2424

Andover

Dr T W I Lovel
The Shepherds Spring Medical
Centre
Cricketers Way
Andover
Hampshire SP10 5DE

0264 61126

Aylesbury

RAF Institute of Pathology &
Tropical Medicine
Halton
Aylesbury
Bucks HP22 5PG

0296 623535

Barking

Dr S N Gupta
7 Salisbury Avenue
Barking
Essex IG11 9XQ

081-594 2023

Barton

Dr D J Sydenham
The Surgery
Hexton Road
Barton
Beds MK45 4TA

0582 882050

Barton Hills

Dr Melville & Partners
Whitehorse Vale, Barton Hills
Luton LU3 4AD

0582 490087

The Surgery
2 Ashdale Gardens, Barton Hills
Luton LU3 4DE

0582 597737

Barrow-in-Furness

Vickers Medical Department
5 Cavendish Park
Barrow-in-Furness
Cumbria LA14 2SE

0229 23366

Barnstaple

(*) The Health Centre
Vicarage Street
Barnstaple
Devon EX32 7BT

0271 71761

Barnsley

(*) The Health Centre
New Street
Barnsley
South Yorks S70 1LP

0226 286122 ext 3100

Basing

Dr J M Fowler
Basing Road (The Hampshire
Clinic)
Basing
Hampshire

0256 472002

Basingstoke

(*) Basingstoke District Hospital
Outpatients Department
Park Prewett
Basingstoke Hants RG24 9IA

0256 473202 Ext 3640 or
0256 71286

Bath

Bath Clinic
Cloverton Dawn Road
Coombe Dawn
Bath
Avon BA2 7BR

0225 835555

Wellcare Health Screening
Centre
7 Monmouth Place
Off Queen Square
Bath BA1 2AU

0225 446220

Beckenham

AMI Sloane Hospital
125 Albemarle Road
Beckenham
Kent BR3 2HS

081-466 6911

Occupational Health Centre
The Wellcome Research
Laboratories
Langley Court
South Eden Park Road
Beckenham
Kent BR3 3BS

081-658 2211

Bedford

Dr J E Hood
Rothesay Surgery
Rothesay House
Rothesay Place
Bedford MK40 3PX

0234 271800

The Surgery
4 De Pary's Avenue
Bedford MK40 2TW

0234 50022/51022

Bicester

The Health Centre
Coker Close
Bicester
Oxon OX6 7AT

0869 249333

Biggleswade
The Surgery
35-37 The Baulk
Biggleswade
Bedfordshire
SG18 0PX

0767 312441

Birmingham

The Medical Room
Birmingham International
Airport
Birmingham B26 3QT

021-767 7136

The Medical Centre
Craig Croft
Chelmsley Wood
Birmingham B37 7TR

021-770 5656

(*) 90 Lancaster Street
Birmingham
B4 7AR

021 235 3428

Drs Massey, Hamilton & Hall
110 Church Lane
Handsworth Wood
Birmingham B20 2ES

021 523 2522

The Surgery
75-77 Cotterills Lane
Alum Rock
Birmingham B8 3EZ

021 327 5111

Blackburn

(*) Larkhill Health Centre
Mount Pleasant
Blackburn BB1 5BJ

0254 63611 ext 231

Blackpool

The Surgery
155 Newton Drive
Blackpool FY3 8LZ

0253 32814

Bletchley

Water Eaton Health Centre
Fern Grove
Bletchley
Bucks

0908 71318

Boston

The Surgery
Main Road
Stickney
Boston
Lincs PE22 8AA

0205 480237

Bolton

Newlands Medical Centre
Chorley New Road
Bolton BL1 5BP

0204 40342/3

Bournemouth

(*) Winton Health Centre
Alma Road
Winton
Bournemouth
Dorset BH9 1BP

0202 519491

The Surgery
1628 Wimbourne Road
Kinson
Bournemouth
Dorset BH11 9AH

0202 573947

Bradford

(*) Leeds Road Hospital
Leeds Road
Bradford

West Yorks BD3 9LH

0274 729681 ext 45/58

Brentwood

The Tile House
33 Shenfield Road
Brentwood
Essex CM15 8AQ

0277 22771

BA Travel Centre
The Surgery
Mount Avenue
Shenfield
Essex CM13 2NL

0277 200169

Brighton

(*) School Clinic
Morley Street
Brighton BN2 2RH

0273 693600 ext 271

Yellow Fever

The Manor Laboratory for
Clinical Pathology
26 New Church Road
Hove BN3 4FH

0273 27363

Bristol

(*) Manulife House
10 Marlborough Street
Bristol BS1 3NP

0272 290666 ext 250

Travel Medical Centre Ltd
Charlotte Keel Health Centre
Seymour Road
Bristol BS5 0UA

0272 354447

Wellperson Health Services
155 Whiteliades Road
Bristol BS8 2RF

0272 238203

The Broadmead Clinic
18 Merchant Street
Bristol BS1 3ET

0272 252552

Broadstairs

Reading Road Surgery
235 Beacon Road
Broadstairs
Kent CT10 3DY

0843 61884

Bromley

Dr G Ladd
Dysart House
13 Ravensbourne Road
Bromley BR1 1HN

081-464 4138

Brough

The Surgery
60 Welton Road
Brough
North Humberside HU15 1BH

Bushey Heath

The Surgery
Rutherford Way
Bushey Heath
Herts WD2 1NJ

081-953 1008

Camberley

Dr Hey
The Surgery
143 Park Road
Camberley
Surrey GU15 2NN

0276 26171

Cambridge

(*) Addenbrooke's Hospital
Hills Road
Cambridge CB2 2QQ

0223 245151 ext 7538

Canterbury

The Chaucer Hospital
Nackington Road
Canterbury
Kent CT4 7AR

0227 455466

Carlisle

(*) The Central Clinic
Victoria Place
Carlisle CA1 1HN

0228 36451

Carterton (Oxfordshire)

The Surgery
17 Alvescot Road
Carterton
Oxfordshire OX8 3JL

0993 844567

Cheadle

AMI Alexandra Hospital
Mill Lane
Cheadle
Cheshire SK8 2PX

061-428 3656

Chelmsford

(*) The Medical Centre
Ground Floor Block A
County hall Chelmsford
Essex CM1 1LX

0245 492211 ext 2756

Cheltenham

Windrush Medical Centre
Laverham House
77 St George's Place
Cheltenham
Glos GL50 3PP

0242 221105

The Surgery
Bakery Crescent
St George's Place
Cheltenham
Glos GL50 3PN

0242 226336

Chesterfield

The Health Centre Saltergate
Chesterfield
Derbyshire S40 1SY

0246 202211

Chipping Norton

West Street Surgery
12 West Street
Chipping Norton
Oxon OX7 5AA

0608 2529

Chislehurst

Dr R W May
The Surgery
42 High Street
Chislehurst Kent BR7 5AX

081-467 5551

Yellow Fever

Chorley Wood

The Elms Surgery
7 Lower Road
Chorley Wood
Herts WD3 5EA

092 78 2468

Cirencester

The Surgery
45 Dollar Street
Cirencester
Gloucestershire GL7 2AU

0285 654733

Dr C M Marriott
1 The Avenue
Cirencester
Gloucestershire GL7 1EH

0285 653122 or 652944

Clacton-on-Sea

Dr G A Sweeney
Ranworth
103 Pier Avenue
Clacton-on-Sea CO15 1NJ

0255 421344

Claygate (Surrey)

Dr R Leary
17 Torrington Road
Claygate
Surrey KT10 0SA

0372 62501

Colchester

Priory House
St Botolph's Street
Colchester
Essex CO2 7EA

0206 560050

The Surgery
Birch
Colchester
Essex CO2 0NL

0206 330222

Corsham

Dr R C F Drummond
The Porch
Corsham
Wilts SN13 0EY

0249 713019

Coventry

(*) Hillsfield Health Centre
1 Howard Street
Coventry CV1 4GH

0203 224055 ext 6035/6036

Crewe

Moss Lane Surgery
Moss Lane
Madeley near Crewe
Cheshire CW3 9NQ

0270 760274

Immunisation against Infectious Disease

Dr B S Tate
Hungerford Road Surgery
Crewe
Cheshire CW1 1EQ

0207 582589

Croydon

Executive Medical Centre
Canterbury House
Sydenham Road
Croydon
Surrey CRO 2LS

081-688 3430

Dagenham

Occupational Health Department
Rhone-Poulenc Ltd
Rainham Road South
Dagenham
Essex RM10 7 XS

081-592 3060

Deal

Dr N J Sharvill
1 Victoria Road
Deal
Kent CT14 7Au

0304 373444

Derby

(*) The Clinic
Cathedral Road
Derby DE1 3PE

0332 45934

Doncaster

(*) The Health Clinic
Chequer Road
Doncaster DN1 2PW

0302 367051 ext 251

Dunstable

The Health Centre
Priory Gardens
Church Street
Dunstable

0582 699622

East Grinstead

The Practice
Judges Close
East Grinstead
Sussex RH19 3AR

0342 24628

Edgware (Middlesex)

Dr C D Korn
104a Stag Lane
Edgware
Middlesex HA8 5LW

081-204 1237

Elstree

Schopwick Surgery
Everett Court
Romeland
Elstree
Herts WD6 3BJ

081-953 1008

Yellow Fever

Enfield

Dr M Gocman
Abernethy
70 Silver Street
Enfield
Middlesex EN1 3EB

081-366 1314

Eagle House Surgery
291 High Street
Enfield
Middlesex EN3 4DN

081-805 4800

Esher

Littleton Surgery
33 Esher Park Avenue
Esher
Surrey KT10 9NY

0372 62235

Exeter

(*) Yellow Fever Vaccination
Clinic
Dean Clarke House
Southernhay East
Exeter EX1 1PQ

0392 411222 ext 6146

Farnborough

Summerlands Surgery
Starts Hill Road
Farnborough
Kent BR6 7AR

0689 52165/61098

Felixstowe

Dr B M G Clarke
Central Surgery
201 Hamilton Road
Felixstowe
Suffolk IP11 7DT

0394 283197

Gateshead

Glenpark Medical Centre
Ravensworth Road
Durston
Gateshead NE11 9AD

091 460 4300

Gatwick

British Airways Vaccination
Centre
North Terminal
London (Gatwick) Airport
Crawley
Sussex RH10 2FH

0293 665444 or 662344

Dr P J C Chapman
Airport Medical Services
Penta Hotel Medical Suite
Gatwick Airport
Horley
Surrey RH6 0BE

0293 776996/820169

Gatwick Medical Services
South Terminal Medical Centre
(3rd Floor)
London (Gatwick) Airport
West Sussex RH6 0NP

0293 507400

Dr M Glanfield
Dan Air Services Ltd
Newman House
Victoria Road
Horley
Surrey RH6 7QC

0293 820700

Civil Aviation Authority
Safety Regulation Group
(Medical Division)
Aviation House, South Area
Gatwick Airport
West Sussex RH6 0YR

0293 567171

Glossop

Peck Health Vaccination Centre
Manor Street
Glossop
Derbyshire SK13 7PS

04574 60860

Gloucester

(*) Gloucestershire Royal
Hospital
Great Western Road
Gloucester GL1 3NN

0452 28555 ext 4210

Dowty Rotol Ltd
Cheltenham Road
Gloucester GL2 9QH

0452 712424

Dr R P Norwich
The Clinic
19 College Green
Gloucester GL1 2ER

Gravesend

The Surgery
30 Old Road West
Gravesend
Kent DA11 0LL

0474 352075

Grays

Dr A J Rigg-Milner
The Surgery
111 Orsett Road
Grays
Essex RM17 5HA

0375 372135/376088

Great Missenden

Chiltern Hospital
Great Missenden
Buckinghamshire HP16 0EN

02406 6565

Yellow Fever

Great Yarmouth

North Sea Medical Centre Ltd
3 Lowestoft Road
Gorleston-on-Sea
Great Yarmouth
Norfolk NR31 6SG

0493 600011/663264

Grimsby

(*) The Clinic
34 Dudley Street
Grimsby
South Humberside DN31 1QQ
0472 74111 ext 7890/7843

Guildford

Robens Institute
Occupational Health Service
30 Occam Road
University of Surrey
Guildford GU2 5YW

0483 68637/68673

Haddenham

Haddenham Health Centre
Banks Road
Haddenham
Bucks HP17 8EE

0844 291874

Harlow

Harlow Industrial Health Service
Edinburgh House,
Edinburgh Way
Harlow
Essex CM20 2DG

0279 22377

Harpenden

Dr D P Tominey
3 Thompson's Close
Harpenden
Herts AL5 4ES

05827 65266

Harrow

Harrow Health Care Centre
84-88 Pinner Road
Harrow
Middlesex HA1 4LF

081-861 1221

Hatfield

Lister House
The Common
Hatfield
Herts AL10 0NL

07072 68811

Heathrow

British Airways Medical Service
Speedbird House Medical Centre
London (Heathrow) Airport
Hounslow
Middlesex TW6 2JA

081-562 5453

British Airways Medical Service
Central Area (Queen's Building)
London (Heathrow) Airport
Hounslow
Middlesex TW6 2BX

081-562 7903

Heathrow Airport Ltd
Queen's Building Medical Centre
Heathrow Airport
Hounslow
Middlesex TW6 1JH

081-745 7187

Hemel Hempstead

Dr Toorawa
Lincoln House Surgery
Wolsey Road
Hemel Hempstead
Herts HP2 4SH

0442 56731

BP Oil UK Ltd.,
BP House
Breakspear Road
Hemel Hempstead
Herts HP2 4UL

0442 225368

Henley-on-Thames

Dr Melhuish
The New Surgery
York Road
Henley-on-Thames
Oxon RG9 2DR

0491 572261

Hereford

Dr. P J Matthews
The Surgery
Moorfield House
Hereford

0432 272175

Hoddesdon

The Health Centre
High Street
Hoddesdon
Herts EN11 8BE

0992 464533

Hornchurch

Marylands
Hornchurch Road
Hornchurch
Essex RM12 4TP

04024 76411

Dr R E Farrow
The Surgery
58B Billet Lane
Hornchurch
Essex RM11 1XY

04024 40187/42377/76113

Yellow Fever

Hounslow

Dr B S Mangat
The Surgery
5 Cecil Road
Hounslow
Middlesex TW3 1NU

081-572 2536

Hull

Dr K J Kutte
415 Beverley Road
Kingston-upon-Hull HU5 1LX

0482 42808

University Health Service
University of Hull
187 Cottingham Road
Kingston-upon-Hull HU5 2EG

0482 46311

(*) The Central Clinic
74 Beverley Road
Kingston-upon-Hull HU3 1YD

0482 223191 ext 2272/2274

Medicos Ltd
Medicos House
79 Beverley Road
Kingston-upon-Hull HU3 1XR

0482 20243

Ilford

The Surgery
150 Longwood Gardens
Clayhall
Ilford
Essex IGE 0BE

081-550 6362

The Roding Hospital
Roding Lane South
Ilford
Essex IG4 5PS

081-551 1100

Ipswich

Orchard Street Health Centre
Ipswich
Suffolk IP4 2PU

0473 213261

King's Lynn

Pott Row Surgery
17 Back Lane
Pott Row
King's Lynn
Norfolk PE32 1BT

0485 600341

Kingston-on-Thames
Dr W Russell
The Surgery
3 Upper Teddington Road
Hampton Wick
Kingston-on-Thames
Surrey KT1 4DL

01-977 2638

The Surgery
14 Fairfield South
Kingston-on-Thames
Surrey KT1 2UJ

081-546 1771

Lancaster

(*) Ashton Road Clinic
Lancaster
Lancs LA4 4RR

0524 65944 ext 3717

Cleveland Medical
Laboratories Ltd
Lancaster and Lakeland Nuffield
Hospital
Meadowside
Lancaster
LA1 3RH

0524 36550/62345 ext 207

Leamington Spa

Croft Medical Centre
Calder Walk
Leamington Spa
Warwickshire CV31 1SA

0926 421153

Leeds

(*) Halton Clinic
2 Primrose Lane, Off Selby Road
Leeds 15
0532 486351

Leicester

(*) St Peter's Health Centre
Sparkenhoe Street
Leicester LE2 0TA

0533 559600 ext 230

BA Travel Centre
16 High Street
Leicester LE1 5YN

0533 516564

Letchworth

Birchwood Surgery
232-240 Nevells Road
Letchworth
Herts SG6 4UB

0462 683456

Lincoln

(*) Newland Health Centre
Newland
Lincoln LN1 1XP

0522 532321 ext 271

Liverpool

(*) International Vaccination
Clinic
Sefton General Hospital
Smithdown Road
Liverpool L3 5QA

051-733 4020 ext 2202

(*) School of Tropical Medicine
Pembroke Place
Liverpool L3 5QA

051-708 9393

General Council of British
Shipping
Mann Island
Pier Head
Liverpool L3 1DQ

051-236 6031

Dr H Debson
Clinical Pathology
Laboratories Ltd
Marine and Travel Medical
Departments
27 Rodney Street
Liverpool L1 9EH

051 708 6767

London N

Dr S Gibeon
Heathfield Surgery
Lyttleton Road
London N2 0EE

081-455 0165/4968

BUPA Medical Centre
Webb House
210 Pentonville Road
King's Cross
London NW1 9TA

071-278 4651

(*) Vaccination Service
Hospital for Tropical Diseases
4 St Pancras Way
London NW1 0PE

071-387 4411 ext 136/137

Dr W Townsley
North-West London Vaccination
Centre
234 Hendon Way
Hendon
London NW4 3NE

081-202 7272

(*) Occupational Health Unit
Central Middlesex Hospital
Acton Lane
London NW10 7NS

071-965 5733

London W

Glaxo Holdings plc
Clarges House
6-12 Clarges Street
London WIY 8DH

071-493 4060

British Gas plc
59 Bryanston Square
London W1A 2AZ

071-723 7030

Dr M Seear
86 Harley Street
London W1

071-580 3256

Immunisation against Infectious Disease

Dr J Joseph
Amoco Europe Incorporated
48 Wimpole Street
London W1M 7BD

071-935 4357 or 071-486 7876

British Airways Immunisation
Medical Centre
156 Regent Street
London W1R 7HG

071-439 9584/5

Thomas Cook Group Limited
45 Berkeley Street
London W1A 1EB

071-499 4000

Dr C Goodson-Wickes
8 Devonshire Place
London W1N 1PB

071-935 5011

PPP Immunization Centre
99 New Cavendish Street
London W1M 7FQ

071-637 8941

West London Vaccinating Centre
53 Great Cumberland Place
London W1H 7LH

071-262 6456

Dr L Roodyn
7 Wimpole Street
London W1M 7AB

071-323 1555

International Medical Centre
21 Upper Wimpole Street
London W1M 7TA

071-486 3063

The Imaging Centre Ltd
109 Harley Street
London W1N 1DG

071-486 4247

Dr C D Korn
42 Harley Street
London W1N 1AB

071-580 0020

Marks & Spencer plc
47-67 Michael House
Baker Street
London W1A 1DN

071-935 4422

(*) St Mary's Hospital
Praed Street
London W2 1NY

071-725 6666

Dr R Hart
4 Norfolk Place
London W2 1QN

071-723 7891

Yellow Fever

Dr R Ng
British Airways Travel Clinic
9 Little Newport Street
London WC2H 7JJ

071-287 2255/3366

Civil Aviation House
45-49 Kingsway
London WC2B 6TE

071-379 7311

The Surgery
1 Avenue Crescent
London W3 8EW

01-992 0530/1963

Dr S M Drage
Bedford Park Surgery
55 South Parade
Chiswick
London W4 5LH

01-994 0298/3333

Dr R Kathuria
1 Glebe Street
Chiswick
London W4 2BD

01-747 4800

Dr N A Thakran
Chiswick Health Centre
Fishers Lane
Chiswick
London W4 1RX

01-995 8393

Dr N Burbidge
2 Oxford Gardens
Chiswick
London W4 3DW

01-995 4396

Queen Charlotte's Maternity
Hospital
Goldhawk Road
London W6 0XG

01-748 4666

Trailfinders Travel Centre
Medical Advisory Centre
42 Earls Court Road
London W8 6EJ

01-938 3444

Dr G Moses
143 Uxbridge Road
London W12 9RD

01-743 1511

Argyle Surgery
128 Argyle Road
Ealing
London W13 8GR
01-991 2103
London S

Dr M M Ferris
4 Frobisher House
Dolphin Square
London SW1 3LN

071-789 8520

Dr P Dorrington Ward
The Surgery
95a Jermyn Street
London SW1Y 6JE

071-930 2800

Dr I C Perry
19 Clivedon Place
London SW1 8HD

071-730 8045

Medical Department
BP Chemicals Ltd
Belgrave-House
76 Buckingham Palace Road
London SW1W 0SU

071-581 1388

Dr A M Vincent
11 Sloane Court West
London SW3 4TD

071-730 1142

Avicenna Clinic
6 Penywern Road
London SW5 9ST

071-370 7731/2 or 071-373
3196/7

Cromwell Hospital
Cromwell Road
London SW5 0TU

071-370 4233

The Surgery
82 Lillie Road
London SW6 1TN
01-386 9299

Dr G Staight
2a Pelham Street
London SW7 3HU

01-584 6511

Dr J M Critchley
63 Cornwall Gardens
London SW7 4BD

01-937 5362

Dr R Gulati
The Surgery
119 Northcote Road
London SW11 6PW

01-228 6762

The Rowans Surgery
1 Windermere Road
Streatham
London SW16 5HT

01-764 0407/8

(*) Keats Clinic, Keats House
Guys Hospital
St Thomas' Street
London SE1 9RT

071-407 7600 ext 3090

Director of Occupational Health
St Thomas Hospital
London SE1 7EH

071-928 9292

PPP Medical Centre
Emblem House
London Bridge Hospital
27 Tooley Street
London SE1 2PR

071-378 0638

AMI Blackheath Hospital
40-42 Lee Terrace
Blackheath
London SE3 9UD

01-318 7722

The Surgery
105 Bellenden Road
London SE15 4QZ

01-639 9622

London E

Occupational Health Department
The London Hospital
(Whitechapel)
London E1 1BB

071-377 7000

City Health Care Ltd
4-7 Chiswell Street
London EC1Y 4TH

071-638 4988

Mildmay Mission Hospital
Hackney Road
London E2 7NA

071-739 2331

Dr Gill & Partners
23 Lawrence Lane
London EC2V 8DA

071-606 6159

Dr H M J Kindness
65 London Wall
London EC2M 7AD

071-638 3001

Barbican Medical Ltd
No 3 White Lyon Court
The Barbican
London EC2Y 8EA

071-588 3146

Dr Brackenridge & partners
3 Lombard Street
London EC3V 9AL

071-626 6985

Dr Hugh Richards
4 Mitre Court Chambers
4 Old Mitre Court
Fleet Street
London EC4Y 7BP

071-353 4151

The Medical Department
Unilever House
Blackfriars Embankment
London EC4 P4BQ

071-822 6017

Dr G Bulger
The Surgery
153 Hainault Road
Leytonstone
London E11 1DT

Dr J Richardson
Island Health
Units 1 & 2
ASDA Superstore
East Ferry Road
London E14

081-537 2311

Loughborough

The Medical Centre
University of Technology
Loughborough
Leicestershire LE11 3TU

0509 263171

Luton

The Surgery
163 Dunstable Road
Luton LU1 1BW

0582 23553/5

Liverpool Road Health Centre
Liverpool Road
Luton LU1 1HH

0583 31321/413302

Lymington

Dr D D Bodley Scott
Wistaria
St Thomas Street
Lymington
Hampshire SO41 9ZH

Maidstone

(*) Springfield
Sandling Road
Maidstone
Kent ME14 2LU

0622 671411 ext 2726

Malvern

The Surgery
28a Avenue Road
Malvern
Worcs WR14 3BG

0684 574773

Manchester

(*) Manchester Travel Clinic
Alexandra Park Health Centre
2 Whitswood Close
Manchester M16 7AW

061-227 9896

(*) Monsall Hospital
Newton Heath
Manchester M10 8WR

061-205 2393

British Airways
Immunisation Centre
Market Street
Manchester M1 1PU

061-832 3019

Medical Link, Room 109
1st Floor, Tower Block Building
Manchester Airport PLC
Manchester M22 5PA

061-489 3344

Dr I G Donnan
MSF Aviation Ltd
South Side Manchester Airport
Wilmslow
Cheshire SK9 4LL

061-499 1444

Occupational Health Service
University of Manchester
William Kay House
327 Oxford Street
Manchester M13 9PG

061-275 6971

Matlock

Dr MacFarlane
The Practice
8 Imperial Road
Matlock
Derbyshire DE4 3NL

0629 582461

Middlesbrough

(*) West Lane Hospital
Acklam Road
Middlesbrough
Cleveland TS5 4EE

0642 813144 ext 265

Milton Keynes

Milton Keynes Occupational
Health Service Ltd
Whalley Drive
Bletchley
Milton Keynes MK3 6EN

0908 75194/5

Mortimer (Berkshire)

Dr I L C Bray
The Surgery
Mortimer
Berks RG7 3SQ

0734 332436

New Malden

72 Coombe Road
New Malden
Surrey
081-949 4422

Newbury

The Health Centre
Thatcham
Newbury
Berkshire RG13 4HH

0635 67171

Immunisation against Infectious Disease

Newcastle Upon Tyne

(*) Shieldfield Health and Social
Services Centre
4 Clarence Walk (Off Stoddart
Street)
Newcastle upon Tyne NE2 1AL

091-273 8811 ext 22666

Newport Isle of Wight

(*) St Mary's Hospital
Newport
Isle of Wight
0983 524081 ext 4209

Newport Pagnell

The Health Centre
Newport Pagnell
Bucks MK16 8EA

0908 211035

Northampton

(*) The Clinic
67 St Giles Street
Northampton NN1 5DQ

0604 37221 ext 2315

Northwood (Middlesex)

The Surgery
Mount Vernon Hospital
Rickmansworth Road
Northwood
Middlesex

09274 20626 or 28488

Norwich

(*) The Health Centre
West Pottergate
Norwich NR2 4BX

0603 620263

Nottingham

(*) Meadows Health Centre
1 Bridgeway Centre
The Meadows
Nottingham NG2 2JG

0602 415333 ext 209

Occupational Health Service
The Boots Company plc
Station Street
Nottingham NG2 3AA

0602 506255 ext 27

Occupational Health Service
The Boots Company plc
1 Thame Road West
Beeston
Nottingham NG2 3AA

0602 506255 ext 27

(*) AMI Park Hospital
Sherwood Lodge Drive, Arnold
Nottingham NG5 8RX

0602 670670

Yellow Fever

Yellow Fever

Oxford

(*) John Radcliffe Hospital
Level 2 Brown Waiting Area
Headley Way,
Headington
Oxford OX2 6HE

0865 249891 ext 4816

The Jericho Health Centre
Walton Street
Oxford OX2 6NW

0865 311234

Dr Bent Juel-Jensen
University of Oxford
Radcliffe Infirmary
Woodstock Road
Oxford OX2 6HE

0865 270079

Paignton

The Clinic
Midvale Road
Paignton
Devon TQ4 5BD

0803 522762

Penzance

(*) Health Clinic
Bellair
Alverton
Penzance TR18 4TA

0736 62321

Peterborough

Jennes Health Centre
Writtlesey
Nr. Peterborough PE7 4EJ

0733 203601

Pewsey

Dr P D Jenkins
The Surgery
Upavon
Pewsey
Wiltshire SN9 6DZ

0980 630221

Plymouth

(*) Community Health
Department
Scott Hospital
Beacon Park Road
Plymouth PL2 2PQ

0752 550741

Portsmouth

(*) Battenburg Avenue Clinic
North End Portsmouth
Hants PO2 0TA

0705 664235

The Surgery
23 Landport Terrace
Southsea
Hants PO1 2RG

0705 736006

Potters Bar

Parkfield Medical Centre
The Walk
Potters Bar
Herts EN6 1QH

0707 59923

National Institute for Biological
Standards and Control
Blanche Lane
South Mimms
Potters Bar
Herts EN6 3PG

0707 54753/54763

Purley

BA Travel Centre
Clarement House
2 Woodcote Valley Road
Purley
Surrey CR2 3AC

081-763 1372

Radlett

The Red House
124 Watling Street
Radlett
Herts WD7 8HB

09276 5606

(*) Shenley Hospital
Shenley
Radlett
Herts WD7 8H13

09276 5631

Ramsgate

Dr P Attwood
Wideham Avenue
Ramsgate
Kent CD1 8AY

0843 593420

Reading

Chancellor House
Shinfield Road
Reading
Berks RG2 7BW

0734 311696

University Health Centre
Northcott Avenue
Reading
Berks RG2 7HE

0734 874551/2

Redbridge

The Roding Hospital
Roding Lane South
Redbridge
Essex IG4 5PZ

081-551 1100

Richmond (Surrey)

(*) The Clinic
King's Road
Richmond
Surrey TW10 6EF

081-940 9879

Rugby

Central Surgery
Corporation Street
Rugby CV21 3SP

0788 74335

Salisbury

The Surgery
Park Road
Tisbury
Salisbury
Wilts SP3 6FF

0747 870204

Sevenoaks

Dr F D Higgs
Amherst Medical Centre
London Road
Sevenoaks
Kent TN13 2JD

0732 459255

Town Medical Centre
25 London Road
Sevenoaks
Kent TN13 1AR

0732 454545

Sheffield

(*) Mulberry Street
Sheffield S1 2PL

0742 768885 ext 157

Richmond Medical Centre
334 Richmond Road
Sheffield S13 8LY

0742 399291

Dr C Kell
The Practice
394 London Road
Sheffield S2 4NB

0742 551184

Shenfield

The Surgery
Mount Avenue
Shenfield
Essex CM13 2NL

0277 224612

Shrewsbury

(*) Cross Houses Hospital
Shrewsbury
Shropshire SY5 6JN

0743 75242 ext 386

Sittingbourne

The Practice
32 London Road
Sittingbourne
Kent ME10 1ND

0795 72109/72100

Immunisation against Infectious Disease

Skipton

Dyneley House Surgery
Dyneley House
Newmarket Street
Skipton BD23 2HZ

0756 69811

The Practice
49 Otley Street
Skipton
Yorkshire BD23 1ET

0756 69622

Slough

The Nuffield Hospital
Wexham Street
Slough
Berkshire SL3 6NH

02816 2999

Slough Occupational Health
Service
30 Bradford Road
Buckingham Avenue
Slough SL1 4PG

0753 22238

Southall

23 Beaconsfield Road
Southall
Middlesex UB1 1BW

01-574 5943

Southampton

Cunard Steamship Company plc
South Western Houses
Canute Road
Southampton
Hampshire SO9 1ZA

0703 229933 ext 366

General Council of British
Shipping
19-23 Canute Road
Southampton SO1 1FJ

0703 223546

(*) Central Health Clinic
East Park Terrace
Southampton SO9 4WA

0703 634321 ext 235/265

The Aldermoor Health Centre
Aldermoor Close
Southampton SO1 6ST

0703 783111

Shirley Health Centre
Grove Road
Shirley
Southampton SO9 32A

0703 783611

PPP Southampton Medical
Centre
PPP House
37 Commercial Road
Southampton SO1 0GG

0703 639922/3

Immunisation against Infectious Disease

Southborne

Southbourne Surgery
337 Main Road
Southbourne
Emsworth
Hants P10 8JH

0243 372623

Southend-on-Sea

(*) Queensway House
Essex Street
Southend on Sea
Essex SS2 5TD

0702 616322 ext 213

Southsea

The Surgery
23 Landport Terrace
Southsea
Hants PO1 2RG

0705 736006

South Shields

General Council of British
Shipping
Suite 12, Lookson House
112 River Drive
South Shields
Tyne & Wear NE33 1DX
091 456 3172

Stanford Le Hope

Dr S R Barton
The Surgery
37 Southend Road
Stanford Le Hope
Essex SS17 0PQ

0375 673064

Stevenage

The Health Centre
5 Stanmore Road
Stevenage SG1 3QA

0438 361111

St Helens

(*) International Vaccination
Centre
Occupational Health Service
Peasley Cross Wing
St. Helens Hospital
Marshalls Cross Road
St. Helens
Merseyside SQ9 3DA

0744 28879

Stoke-on-Trent

Briches Medical Centre
Diana Road, Briches Head
Stoke-on-Trent
Staffs ST1 6RS

0782 286843

Immunisation against Infectious Disease

Stratford-Upon-Avon

Rother House Medical Centre
Alcester Road
Stratford-upon-Avon CV37 6PP
0789 68249

Sunbury-on-Thames

International Medicine
Unocal Corporation
32 Cadbury Road
Sunbury-on-Thames
Middlesex TW16 7LU

0932 785600

Sunningdale

Dr J McKendrick
Magnolia House
Sunningdale SL5 0QT

0344 20404

Sunninghill

Dr P N Withfield
Kings Corner Surgery
Sunninghall
Ascot
Berks SL5 0AE

0344 23181

Sutton

Dr Latham
The Surgery
54 Bershill Avenue
Sutton SM1 4EB

081-642 8011

Swindon

Dr N J A Theobald
Merchiston
10 Swindon Road
Stratton St Margaret
Swindon
Wilts SN3 4QB

0793 823307

Swindon Private Health Centre
3 Cricklade Court
Cricklade Street
Swindon
Wilts SN1 3EY

0793 513255

Tadley

Holmwood Health Centre
Franklin Avenue
Tadley
Hants RG26 6ER

0734 814166

Taunton

(*) County Hall
Taunton
Somerset TA1 4DY

0823 73491 ext 245/255

Thatcham

The Health Centre
Thatcham
Newbury
Berks RG18 4HH

0635 67171

Immunisation against Infectious Disease

Tilbury

The Health Centre
London Road
Tilbury
Essex RM18 8EB

03752 2028

The Surgery
2 Bure
East Tilbury
Essex RM18 8SF

0375 858657

Tisbury (Wilts)

The Surgery
Park Road
Tisbury
Salisbury
Wilts SP3 6FF

0747 870204

Tonbridge

Dr J M Hawkings
Warders Medical Centre
East Street
Tonbridge
Kent TN9 1LA

Tring

The Surgery
Rothschild House
Chapel Street
Tring
Herts HP23 6PU

044282 2468

Truro

(*) District Health Office
4 St Clements Vean
Tregolls Road
Truro TR1 1NR

0872 72202

Twyford

The Surgery
Loddon Hall Road
Twyford
Berkshire RG10 9JA

0734 340112

Wantage

Dr D J C Flower
Newbury Street Practice
Wantage Health Centre
Garston Lane, Wantage
Oxon OX12 7AY

02357 3451

Research and Development
Centre
Group Technology Department
Metal Box plc
Denchworth Road
Wantage
Oxon ON12 9BP

Immunisation against Infectious Disease

Ware

Dr I H Bridges
Church Street Surgery
St Mary's Courtyard
Church Street
Ware
Herts SG12 9EG

0920 68941

Watford

Coach House Surgery
12 Park Avenue
Watford
Herts WD1 7HP

0923 223178/247745/6

Wellingborough

Medical Centre
106 Gold Street
Wellingborough NN8 4BT

0933 222050

Welwyn Garden City

Group Practice
4 Hall Grove
Welwyn Garden City
Herts AL7 4PL

0707 323355

West Bromwich

Midlands Occupational
Health Service Ltd
83 Birmingham Road
West Bromwich
West Midlands B70 1PX

021-553 7116/9

Westgate on Sea

The Surgery
60 Westgate Bay Avenue
Westgate-on-Sea
Kent CT8 8SN

0843 313335

West Malling

West Malling Group Practice
Milverton
116 High Street
West Malling
Kent ME19 6NE

0732 870212

Weybridge

Weybridge Health Centre
Minorca Road
Weybridge
Surrey KT13 8DU

0932 853366

Yellow Fever

Weymouth

Cross Road Surgery
Cross Road
Weymouth
Dorset

0305 785188

Whitby

Whitby Group Practice
The Health Centre
Whitby Hospital
Whitby
North Yorkshire YO21 1DP

0947 802828

Willenhall

The Surgery
Ednam Hall
63 Bloxwich Road
Willenhall
West Midlands WV13 1AZ

0902 608838

Winchester

Dr J M Flower
The Sarum Road Nursing Home
Sarum Road
Winchester
Hants

0256 472002

Windsor

Dr B Barua
Lee House
84 Osborne Road
Windsor SL4 3EW

0753 861612

Woking

The Health Centre
Hermitage Road
St Johns
Woking
Surrey GU21 1TD

04862 23451

Worcester Park (Surrey)

(*) The Clinic
Manor Drive
Worcester Park
Surrey KT4 7LG

081-337 0246

Yaxley

Yaxley Group Practice
The Health Centre
Lansdowne Road
Yaxley
Peterborough PE7 3JL

0733 240478

York

(*) Monkgate Health Centre
31 Monkgate
York YO3 7PV

0904 30351 ext 19

Immunisation against Infectious Disease

Scotland

Aberdeen

(*) View Terrace Clinic
1 View Terrace
Aberdeen AB2 4RS

0224 631633

Ayrshire

(*) Ayrshire Central Hospital
Irvine KA12 8SS

0294 74191

Dundee

(*) King's Cross Hospital
Clepington Road
Dundee DD3 8EA

0382 816116 ext 224

Edinburgh

(*) 15-17 Carlton Terrace
Edinburgh EH7 5DD

031-557 2100

Lifewatch
Drumsheugh Gardens
Edinburgh EH3 7QJ

031 226 2794/5

Drs Ryecroft & Lacey
The Surgery
84 Main St.,
Davidsons Mains
Edinburgh EH4 5AB

031 336 2291

Glasgow

(*) 20 Cochrane Street
Glasgow G1 1JA

041-227 4411

Lifewatch
5-6 Park Terrace
Glasgow G3

041 332 8010

Orkney

(*) Orkney Health Board
New Scapa Road, Kirkwall
Orkney KW15 1BH

0856 2763 ext 257

Shetland

(*) Gilbert Bain Hospital
Lerwick
Shetland Isles ZE1 0RB

0595 5678

WALES

Cardiff

(*) St David's Hospital
Cowbridge Road East
Cardiff CF1 9TZ

0222 372451 ext 2662/2669

Haverfordwest

(*) Community Health Clinic
Merlins Hill
Haverfordwest
Dyfed SA61 1PG

0437 67801 ext 251

Llandudno

(*) Aberconwy Community Office
Llandudno
Gwynedd LL30 1LB

0492 860011

Newport (Gwent)

(*) Clytha Clinic
Clytha Park Road
Newport
Gwent NP6 4PA

0633 64011

Penarth (S Glam)

Dr E F Griffith
British Shipping Vaccination
Centre
15-16 Station Road
Penarth
S Glamorgan CF6 2EP

0222 702301

Swansea

(*) Swansea Central Clinic
21 Orchard Street
Swansea SA1 1PN

0792 51501 ext 303

Wrexham

Dr P Saul
The Clinic
Beech Avenue
Rhos
Wrexham
Clwyd LL14 1AA

0978 845955

NORTHERN IRELAND

Ballymena

(*) 51 Castle Street
Ballymena
N Ireland

0266 56324/2108/44160

Belfast

(*) The Clinic
Lincoln Avenue
Belfast
N Ireland

0232 748363

Omagh

(*) The Health Centre
Mountjoy Road
Omagh Co Tyrone
N Ireland

0662 3521 ext 263

ISLE OF MAN

Douglas

(*) Noble's Hospital
Douglas
Isle of Man

0624 73661 ext 279

20 Meningococcal infection

20.1 Introduction

20.1.1 Meningococcal meningitis and septicaemia are systemic infections caused by *Neisseria meningitidis*. Meningococci are gram negative diplococci which are divided into antigenetically distinct groups, the commonest of which are B, C, A, Y and W135. They are further subdivided by type and sulphonamide sensitivity.

20.1.2 Group B strains accounted for 61% of all isolates submitted to the Public Health Laboratory Service Meningococcal Reference Laboratory in 1988. Group C strains have risen from 27% in 1984 to 35% in 1988. Group A strains are rare in this country (less than 2%) but are the epidemic strains in other parts of the world.

20.1.3 Irregular upsurges of meningococcal infection occur in the United Kingdom with the previous wave in the mid 1970's. The present upsurge began in 1984 and probably reached its peak in 1988. During the first two weeks of 1988 there were 67 and 66 notifications respectively and there were 1309 notifications of meningococcal meningitis throughout the year with 177 deaths. The incidence of meningococcal disease is highest in infants followed by one to five year olds, but the recent epidemic of Group B 15 P1.16 and the new B4 strain have been associated with an increased incidence in teenagers.

(See Graph ix Page 161)

20.1.4 The carriage rate for all meningococci in the normal population is about 10% although rates vary with age; about 25% of young adults may be carriers at any one time.

20.1.5 Meningococci are transmitted by droplet spread or direct contact from carriers or from individuals in the early stages of the illness; the probable route of invasion is via the nasopharynx. The incubation period is two to three days, and the onset of disease varies from fulminant to insidious with mild prodromal symptoms. Early symptoms and signs are usually malaise, pyrexia and vomiting. Headache, photophobia, drowsiness

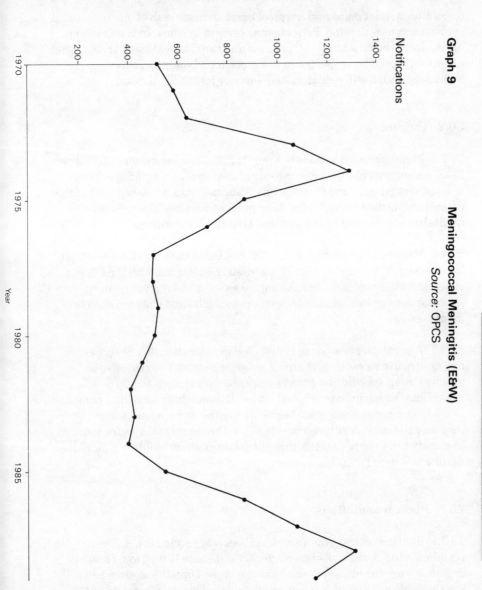

Graph 9

Meningococcal Meningitis (E&W)
Source: OPCS

Notifications

Year

Meningococcal infection

or confusion, joint pains and a typical haemorrhagic rash of meningococcal septicaemia may develop. Patients may present in coma. In young infants particularly, the onset may be insidious and the classical signs absent. The diagnosis should be suspected in the presence of vomiting, pyrexia, irritability and, if still patent, raised anterior fontanelle tension.

20.2 Vaccine

20.2.1 Meningococcal vaccine is a purified, heat stable, lyophilised extract from the polysaccharide outer capsule of *Neisseria meningitidis*, effective against serogroup A and C organisms. Vaccine contains 50mcg each of the respective purified bacterial capsular polysaccharides. **There is no available vaccine effective against Group B organisms**.

20.2.2 Vaccine must be stored at 2-8°C and the diluent must not be frozen. Vaccine should be reconstituted immediately before use with the diluent supplied by the manufacturer. A single dose of 0.5ml is given by deep subcutaneous or intramuscular injection to adults and children from two months of age.

20.2.3 A serological response is detected in more than 90% of recipients and occurs five to seven days after a single injection. The response is strictly Group specific and confers no protection against Group B organisms. Young infants respond less well than adults with little response to the Group C polysaccharide below 18 months and similar lack of response to Group A polysaccharide below three months. Vaccine induced immunity lasts approximately three years; in younger children a more rapid decline in antibody has been noted.

20.3 Recommendations

20.3.1 Routine vaccination with meningococcal vaccine is not recommended as the risk of meningococcal disease is very low, Group B organisms are the major cause of disease in the United Kingdom and a considerable number of cases of meningococcal disease from Group C organisms occur in children too young to be protected with presently available vaccines.

Immunisation against Infectious Disease

20.3.2 **Contacts of cases:** Close contacts of cases of meningococcal meningitis have a considerably increased risk of developing the disease in the subsequent months, despite appropriate chemoprophylaxis. Immediate family or close contacts of cases of Group A or Group C meningitis should be given meningococcal vaccine in addition to chemoprophylaxis. Vaccine should not be given to contacts of Group B cases.

20.3.3 **Local Outbreaks:** In addition to sporadic cases, outbreaks of meningococcal infections from Group C organisms tend to occur in closed or semi-closed communities such as schools and military establishments. Vaccination has been shown to be effective in controlling epidemics, reducing infection rates but not carriage rates. Advice on the use of meningococcal vaccines is available from:-

Communicable Disease Surveillance Centre
(081-200 6868).

Public Health Laboratory Service
Meningococcal Reference Laboratory
(061 445 2416).

Communicable Disease (Scotland) Unit
(041 946 7120).

Meningococcal Reference (Scotland) Laboratory
(041 946 7120).

Meningococcal vaccine has no part to play in the management of outbreaks of Group B meningococcal meningitis.

20.3.4 **Travel:** There are areas of the world where the risk of acquiring meningococcal infection is much higher than in this country particularly for those visitors who live or travel 'rough', such as hitch-hikers or 'trekkers'. These areas include the meningitis belt of Africa where epidemics of Group A infections occur in the dry season, the area of New Delhi, Nepal and Mecca.

The meningitis belt of Africa lies mainly between latitudes 15°N and 5°N except in Uganda and Kenya where it reaches the equator.

Immunisation against Infectious Disease 169

It includes:

a. Southern Sub-Saharan parts of Senegal, Mali, Niger, Chad and Sudan.
b. All of Gambia, Guinea, Togo and Benin.
c. South-West Ethiopia.
d. Northern parts of Sierra Leone, Liberia, Ivory Coast, Nigeria, Cameroon, Central African Republic, Uganda and Kenya.

In the meningitis belt, epidemics have a seasonal character, appearing at the onset of the dry season (December – February) with a peak at the driest period when there is less than 10% relative humidity. Epidemics usually stop with the onset of the rains in May-June.

In 1988 and 1989 Saudi Arabia required vaccination of pilgrims coming to the Haj annual pilgrimage. In 1987, there were 23 cases of Group A meningococcal meningitis in pilgrims from England or their direct contacts; in 1988 only one of 140 pilgrims returning to England carried the epidemic strain.

20.3.5 Meningococcal vaccine may be given to HIV positive individuals in the absence of contraindications.

20.4 Adverse Reactions

20.4.1 Generalised reactions are rare although pyrexia occurs more frequently in young children than in adults.

20.4.2 Injection site reactions occur in approximately 10% of recipients and last for approximately 24-48 hours.

20.4.3 All adverse reactions should be reported to the Committee on Safety of Medicines using the yellow card system.

20.5 Contraindications

20.5.1 Vaccination should be postponed in individuals suffering from an acute febrile illness.

Immunisation against Infectious Disease

20.5.2 Although there is no information to suggest that meningococcal vaccine is unsafe during pregnancy, it should only be given when this is unavoidable, i.e. required for travel. During an epidemic of meningococcal meningitis in Brazil, no adverse events were reported in pregnant women receiving vaccine.

20.6 Supplies

20.6.1 The following meningococcal vaccines are licensed and available:-

Meningivac (A+C), Merieux UK Ltd 0628 785291

ACVax, Smith, Kline and French 0707 325111

20.7 Bibliography

The epidemiology and control of meningococcal disease.
Communicable Disease Report 1989 89/08.

Antibody response to serogroup A and C polysaccharide vaccines in infants born to mothers vaccinated during pregancy.
McCormick J B, Gusman H H et al.
J of Clin. Investigation, 1980;65: 1141-1144.

Meningococcus Group A vaccine in children three months to five years of age. Adverse reactions and immunogenicity related to endotoxin content and molecular weight of the polysaccharide.
Peltola H, Kayhty H, Kuronen T, Haque N, Sanna S, Makela P H.
J. Pediatr. 1978; 92: 818-882.

Kinetics of antibody production to Group A and Group C meningococcal polysaccharide vaccines administered during the first six years of life; prospects for routine immunisation of infants and children.
Gold R, Lepow M L, Goldschneider I, Draper T F, Gotschlich E C.
J Infect Dis 1979; 140: 690-7.

Control of Meningococcal Disease.
Jones D M.
BMJ 1989; 292: 542-543.

Secondary cases of meningococcal infection among close family and
household contacts in England and Wales, 1984-7.
Cooke R P D, Riordan T, Jones D M, Painter M J.
BMJ 1989; 298: 555-558.

21 Varicella/Herpes Zoster

21.1 Introduction

21.1.1 Varicella (chickenpox) is an acute highly infectious disease which is transmitted directly by personal contact or droplet spread, and indirectly via fomites. In the home the secondary infection rate from a case of chickenpox can be as high as 90%. It is most common in children below the age of ten in whom it is usually mild. Vesicles appear without prodromal illness on the face and scalp, spreading to the trunk and abdomen and eventually to the limbs; after three or four days they dry with granular scabs and are usually followed by further crops. Vesicles may be so few as to be missed or so numerous that they become confluent, covering most of the body. The disease can be more serious in adults, particularly for pregnant women; for neonates and immunosuppressed individuals the risk is greatly increased (21.1.4, 21.1.5).

The incidence is seasonal and reaches a peak from March to May. The incubation period is between two and three weeks. Virus is plentiful in the naso-pharynx in the first few days and in the vesicles before they dry up; the infectious period is therefore from one to two days before the rash appears until the vesicles are dry. This may be prolonged in immunosuppressed patients.

21.1.2 Herpes zoster is caused by the reactivation of the patient's varicella virus. It is transmissible to susceptible individuals as chickenpox but there is very little evidence that it can be acquired from another individual with chickenpox. Although more common in the elderly, it can occur in children and especially in immunosuppressed individuals. Vesicles appear in the dermatome representing cranial or spinal ganglia where the virus has been dormant. The affected area may be intensely painful with associated paraesthesia.

21.1.3 Since chickenpox is so common in childhood, 90% of adults are immune. However when it occurs in adults, it carries a risk of fulminating varicella pneumonia which can be rapidly fatal. This risk may be higher in pregnant women who should therefore be closely observed and admitted to hospital if necessary so that their condition can be monitored and they

Immunisation against Infectious Disease

173

Varicella/Herpes Zoster

can be treated promptly with acyclovir.

21.1.4 Risks to the fetus and neonate from maternal chickenpox are related to the time of infection in the mother:-

a. In the first five months of pregnancy:- Congenital varicella syndrome includes major abnormalities of most organs leading to abortion or neonatal death. From a number of studies the incidence has been variously estimated at 2-5% of those infected in the first four months of pregnancy.

b. In the 2nd and 3rd trimesters of pregnancy:- Asymptomatic congenital infection presenting later as herpes zoster in an otherwise healthy child with no history of chicken pox.

c. A week before to a week after delivery:- Severe and even fatal disease in the neonate. Although the risk decreases after this period it remains higher than in older children and half the deaths under one year occur during the first month of life.

21.1.5 The risk of severe or fatal varicella/zoster is increased in the following:-

a. Immunosuppressed individuals in whom mortality is high from disseminated infection or encephalitis.

b. Individuals with debilitating disease in whom normal immunological mechanisms may be impaired.

21.2 Varicella vaccine

Live attenuated varicella vaccine is in the process of development, but currently no vaccine is licensed for use in the UK.

21.3 Human Varicella-zoster immunoglobulin (VZIG)

This is made from UK donors by Blood Products Laboratory, distributed by the Public Health Laboratory Service (21.8) and in Scotland, by the Blood

Varicella/Herpes Zoster

Immunisation against Infectious Disease

Transfusion Service. It is prepared from pooled plasma of blood donors with a history of recent chickenpox or herpes zoster, or from those who on screening are found to have suitably high titres of V-Z antibody. The V-Z antibody content of each batch is titrated and is substantially higher than that in normal immunoglobulin. The supply of VZIG is limited by the availability of suitable donors and its use is therefore restricted to those at greatest risk and for whom there is evidence that it is effective.

21.3.1 VZIG is supplied in ampoules containing 250mg protein in 1.7ml of fluid with added thiomersal and sodium chloride.

21.3.2 It should be stored in a refrigerator between 2-8°C. Under these conditions it has a shelf life of three years. It can be stored for short periods at room temperature; it must NOT be frozen.

21.3.3 All immunoglobulins are prepared from HIV negative donors.

21.4 Recommendations

Because of the increased risk of serious disease, VZIG is recommended for individuals in contact with chickenpox or herpes zoster in the following groups.

21.4.1 **Immunosuppressed patients who within three months of the contact have been on high-dose steroids (eg 2mg/kg/day of prednisolone for more than a week).**

Whenever possible, patients in contact who are without a **definite** history of chickenpox should be screened for varicella/zoster (V-Z) antibody (21.7); only those WITHOUT antibody require VZIG. In an emergency, antibody can be estimated within 24 hours; VZIG can be ordered (see 21.8) and returned if the test is positive.

21.4.2 **Bone-marrow transplant recipients**

Following contact with chickenpox or herpes zoster, these patients should be given VZIG **despite a history of chickenpox.**

NOTE: all patients on long-term immunosuppressive treatment (such as those following transplant) should be screened for V-Z antibody. Many will have antibody, among them some with a negative history of chickenpox.

21.4.3 Individuals with debilitating disease

These should be treated as in 21.4.1.

21.4.4 Neonates

VZIG is recommended for the following:-

a. Those whose mothers develop chickenpox (but not zoster) in the period seven days before to one month after delivery.

b. Those in contact with chickenpox or zoster whose mothers have no history of chickenpox or who on testing have no antibody.

c. Those in contact with chickenpox who are born before 30 weeks of gestation or with a birth weight less than 1kg; these may not possess maternal antibody despite a positive history in the mother.

The following do NOT require VZIG since maternal antibody will be present:-

d. Infants born more than seven days after the onset of maternal chickenpox.

e. Infants whose mothers have a positive history of chickenpox and/or a positive antibody result.

f. Infants whose mothers develop zoster before or after delivery.

NOTE: Neonatal varicella can still develop in infants who have received VZIG. About two thirds of infants, whose mothers develop chickenpox around the time of delivery, develop chickenpox. This is usually mild but rarely, fatal cases have occurred.

21.4.5 Pregnant women

All pregnant contacts of chickenpox without a **definite** history of chickenpox should be tested for V-Z antibody before VZIG is given since about two-thirds of women have antibody despite a negative history of chickenpox. Only those WITHOUT antibody require VZIG.

NOTE: VZIG does not prevent infection even when given within 72 hours of exposure. However when given up to ten days after exposure it may attenuate the disease in pregnant women (21.1.4).

21.4.6 Since VZIG does not prevent infection it is not given to pregnant women with the intention of preventing congenital varicella syndrome. When supplies of VZIG are short it may not be possible to issue it for pregnant contacts of chickenpox.

21.5 HIV positive individuals

(i) Asymptomatic HIV positive individuals do NOT require VZIG after contact with chickenpox since there is no evidence of increased risk of serious illness in these individuals.

(ii) HIV positive individuals with symptoms should be given VZIG after contact with chickenpox without antibody testing if they have no history of chickenpox or are known to be V-Z antibody negative.

21.6 Dose of VZIG for prophylaxis

0 - 5 years	250 mg
6 - 10 years	500 mg
11 - 14 years	750 mg
15 -	1000 mg

This is given by **intramuscular** injection as soon as possible and not later than ten days after exposure. It must NOT be given intravenously.

If a second exposure occurs after three weeks, a further dose is required.

21.7 Treatment

There is no evidence that VZIG is effective in the treatment of severe disease. However, since antibody production can be delayed in immunosuppressed individuals, intravenous commercial preparations of normal human immunoglobulin may be used to provide an immediate source of antibody.

21.8 Supplies

VZIG is made by Blood Products Laboratory (Tel. 081 953 6191) and distributed by all Public Health Laboratories and by Communicable Disease Surveillance Centre (CDSC) (Tel. 081 200 6868).

Scotland: Blood Transfusion Service.
Northern Ireland: The Laboratories, Belfast City Hospital
Tel. 0232 323241

No commercial preparation of VZIG is available.

21.9 VZIG is well tolerated. Very rarely anaphylactoid reactions occur in individuals with hypogammaglobulinaemia who have IgA antibodies, or those who have had an atypical reaction to blood transfusion.

21.10 Severe reactions should be reported to the Committee on Safety of Medicines using the yellow card system.

21.11 Management of hospital outbreaks

21.11.1 Susceptible staff exposed to chickenpox should whenever possible be excluded from contact with high risk patients from eight to 21 days after exposure to a case of chickenpox or zoster.

21.11.2 It is recommended that hospital staff without a definite history of chickenpox should be routinely screened for V-Z antibody so that those

Immunisation against Infectious Disease

susceptible are already identified. This is particularly important for staff in contact with high risk groups such as pregnant women and immunosuppressed patients.

21.12 For advice on testing for V-Z antibody, contact local Public Health or Hospital Laboratory.

22 Appendix 1

Japanese B Encephalitis

Japanese B encephalitis occurs throughout South East Asia and the Far East, predominantly during the monsoon season. The disease is transmitted to man by the bite of a calicine mosquito that dwells in rice-fields. Vaccination should be considered for visitors during the monsoon to rural areas, particularly where rice growing and pig farming co-exist. Short visits (for less than two weeks) which avoid these risk elements, do not generally indicate need for vaccination.

An inactivated vaccine is available in the UK on a named-patient basis from Cambridge Selfcare Diagnostics Limited (Telephone 091 261 5950). A primary course of two 1ml injections (SC) administered 7-14 days apart gives protection for a year. Full immunity however then takes a month or more to develop. A single reinforcing dose should be given after a year. A high degree of protection is achieved by an initial course of three doses, the third dose being given a month after primary vaccination.

Tick Borne Encephalitis

This disease is caused by a virus transmitted to man by the bite of an infected tick. Warm forested parts of Europe and Scandinavia, especially where there is heavy undergrowth, give the greatest risk in late spring and summer. Those walking or camping in such areas should wear clothing that covers most skin surface and use insect repellents on socks and outer clothes.

A killed vaccine is available on a named-patient basis from Immuno Limited (Telephone 0732-458101) and should be used where prolonged exposure is likely in those who work, camp or walk the risk areas. The full primary course consists of three injections of 0.5ml (given IM) the second 4-12 weeks later and the third 9-12 months after the second dose. Protection then lasts three years or more and may be reinforced within a period of six years by a single dose. A shorter primary course of two injections gives protection for one year.

Immunisation against Infectious Disease

23 Appendix II

Rapid schedule for travellers

When required to travel abroad at short notice, or when insufficient time
remains before travelling to undertake a full programme of vaccines, a
rapid schedule may have to be used to achieve the best protection in the
available time. Whenever possible, the recommended intervals between
doses and between vaccines should be followed. Not all of the following
vaccines are needed by all travellers and the schedule should be adopted
for individuals' needs and in accordance with the requirements for the
countries to be visited.

DAY 1	Cholera	1st dose
	Typhoid	1st dose
	Tetanus	1st dose
	Oral Polio	1st dose
DAY 5	Yellow Fever	
DAY 13	Cholera	2nd dose
	Oral Polio	2nd dose
	Typhoid	2nd dose
DAY 28	Tetanus	2nd dose
	Oral polio	3rd dose - see 7.5.4
	Immunoglobulin	1st dose

This schedule only provides two doses of tetanus and the course will need
to be completed following the traveller's return.

Printed in UK for HMSO Dd 292951 C1570 5/90 (43311)

Appendix II